Genetics and Mental Illness

Evolving Issues for Research and Society

Edited by

Laura Lee Hall

National Alliance for the Mentally Ill
Arlington, Virginia

Plenum Press • New York and London

Library of Congress Cataloging-in-Publication Data

Genetics and mental illness : evolving issues for research and society
    edited by Laura Lee Hall.
        p.   cm.
    Includes bibliographical references and index.
    ISBN 0-306-45166-2
    1. Mental illness--Genetic aspects.   I. Hall, Laura Lee.
    [DNLM: 1. Mental Disorders--genetics.   WM 140 G328 1996]
  RC455.4.G4G438   1996
  616.89'042--dc20
  DNLM/DLC
  for Library of Congress   95-50379
                                                                   CIP

ISBN 0-306-45166-2

© 1996 Plenum Press, New York
A Division of Plenum Publishing Corporation
233 Spring Street, New York, N. Y. 10013

Printed in the United States of America

To my parents Monk and Betty Hall.
They have nurtured my growth and development,
as a person and professional.
I am lucky to have so much love
in my gene pool.

Contributors

Mary Ann Beall Virginia Alliance for the Mentally Ill, Richmond, Virginia 23215

Robert Mullan Cook-Deegan National Academy of Sciences, Washington, D.C. 20418

Stephen V. Faraone Harvard Institute of Psychiatric Epidemiology and Genetics; Harvard Medical School Department of Psychiatry at the Massachusetts Mental Health Center and Brockton/West Roxbury VA Medical Center; and Pediatric Psychopharmacology Unit, Psychiatry Service, Massachusetts General Hospital, Boston, Massachusetts 02114

Irving I. Gottesman Department of Psychology, University of Virginia, Charlottesville, Virginia 22903

Laura Lee Hall National Alliance for the Mentally Ill, Arlington, Virginia 22203

Kay Redfield Jamison Department of Psychiatry, Johns Hopkins School of Medicine, Baltimore, Maryland 21218

Janet E. Johnson Department of Psychiatry, Columbia University, College of Physicians & Surgeons, New York, New York 10032

Charles A. Kaufmann Department of Psychiatry, Columbia University, College of Physicians & Surgeons, New York, New York 10032

Herbert Pardes Department of Psychiatry, Columbia University, College of Physicians & Surgeons, New York, New York 10032

Robert Plomin Institute of Psychiatry, London SE5 8AF, United Kingdom

Ming T. Tsuang   Harvard Institute of Psychiatric Epidemiology and Genetics; Harvard Medical School Department of Psychiatry at the Massachusetts Mental Health Center and Brockton/West Roxbury VA Medical Center; and Department of Epidemiology, Harvard School of
Public Health, Boston, Massachusetts 02115

Preface

I was christened into the world of psychiatric genetics more than four years ago. At the time, I was preparing a report to the U.S. Congress on the status of biological research into severe mental illnesses. What I found was a bloody battlefield of ideology and ambition. Antipsychiatry and anti-science demagogues, though small in number and dwindling, denounced, ridiculed, and denied that genes played any role in severe mental illnesses, some denying the reality of these illnesses altogether. At the other extreme, some scientists pressed ahead to find THE schizophrenia gene. The revolution in molecular biology inspired these scientists; major newspapers celebrated their early, but often short-lived, successes.

Unfortunately, these polemics obscured the mountains of data documenting the genetic underpinnings of schizophrenia and other such brain diseases. Genes clearly play a role in these illnesses. But genes are not the sole culprit, and no one gene is likely to be the sole progenitor.

The clear and convincing data were not the only things lost in the heat of the psychiatric gene wars. The implications of our scientific findings have been all but ignored. As time was wasted debating the reality of mental illness and whether genes are all or nothing in these conditions, we neglected some of the real questions that emerge from this science: questions about what these data mean to people with severe mental illnesses and their families, about how clinicians will relay incomplete and complicated data, and about how society will use this information—to help individuals with these illnesses or to further denigrate and discriminate against them. Indeed, the controversies plaguing psychiatric genetics have to some extent kept our nation's leading institution of human genetics research and analysis—the National Center for Human Genome Research and its arm examining ethical and societal issues—from considering mental illnesses at all.

Being a person committed to improving the treatment and understanding of severe mental illnesses and, at heart, a pragmatist, I wanted to prepare a book on psychiatric genetics, minus the rhetoric. I wanted to give interested clinicians, researchers, and informed laypersons a sense of the impressive array of data gathered to date in this field. I also wanted to engage a fresh discussion of what these data mean to people with mental illnesses, their families, and our society. So I persuaded some of my friends and colleagues to prepare papers on this topic—summarizing data and exploring its implications.

This book is the result of our work. It summarizes our knowledge about the genetics of severe mental illnesses. It relays the unsteady and unpredictable ascent that typifies the endeavor we call scientific research. It applies the knowledge base of medical genetics to psychiatric genetics. It asks new questions about the meaning of these data to people with severe mental illnesses and their family members. And it challenges us, as a society, to be thoughtful and humane in the application of new knowledge.

I hope this book sheds more light than heat.

In addition to the contributing authors—who are all not only extremely intelligent, but also generous with their time and effective in their communication—I want to acknowledge Drs. Neil Risch and E. Fuller Torrey for the many hours of conversation about the complicated subject of this book. They have all taught me a great deal. These extremely knowledgeable individuals stand out as committed both to scientific rigor and to people with severe mental illnesses.

Laura Lee Hall

Contents

CHAPTER 1

Introduction

LAURA LEE HALL

A few short years after modern genetics announced the spoil of its first successful gene hunt—the location of the Huntington disease gene—psychiatric genetics embraced these techniques, fielding gene hunts of its own and touting successful gene finds. Many researchers joined the effort. Leaders in the field proclaimed the ultimate clinical importance of this research. Newspapers heralded the new age.

The early clamor around psychiatric genetics also sowed the seeds of a backlash. Naysayers dismissed the importance of genes in major mental disorders. Alarmists sounded bells of potential abuse. Scientific research fell into the very trap it laid: Early gene-hunt successes proved difficult to replicate and some findings were retracted.

It is difficult to maneuver on this landscape of controversy and contradictions. Little light has radiated from the heated battlefield of psychiatric genetics. What sound information can clinicians, people with mental disorders, and their family members extract from the hullabaloo? What is the truth about psychiatric genetics?

The absence of straight, sober talk about psychiatric genetics is not a reflection of false or failed science. Rather, it is the complexity of this research endeavor, the very complexity of genetic inputs to mental illness, filtered through polarizing lens, that has confounded understanding. Many types and sources of data document the heritability of severe mental illnesses like schizophrenia and manic-depression. The research is not complete; the plot has yet to completely unravel. Genes are not the entire story,

LAURA LEE HALL • National Alliance for the Mentally Ill, Arlington, Virginia 22203.

Genetics and Mental Illness: Evolving Issues for Research and Society, edited by Laura Lee Hall. Plenum Press, New York, 1996.

but they are important players. What is more, the data we have right now can—*should*—be available in the clinical setting. And we need to start thinking about what this research means to our society, now and in the future.

This collection of essays seeks to present straight, sober talk about psychiatric genetics. Leading researchers present the facts as well as the theoretical backdrop for modern psychiatric genetics. Policy analysts and a consumer/family member discuss what this means to our society. What this book hopefully presents are scientifically accurate and humanly important discussions of psychiatric genetics.

The volume begins with an overview of trends in psychiatric genetic research, prepared by Charles A. Kaufmann, Janet E. Johnson, and Herbert Pardes. These leaders in psychiatry and genetics rightly acknowledge the profound impact of modern genetics on clinical medicine at large. Even as techniques of molecular genetics have revealed genes for cystic fibrosis, diabetes mellitus, breast cancer, and other diseases, its application to psychiatric illnesses has produced confusing results. While genes linked to Alzheimer's disease have been identified and potential genetic loci for manic-depression and schizophrenia revealed, by and large psychiatric genetics has produced ambivalent results. Future progress and research direction can best be understood, according to the authors, in terms of complex models for mental illness inheritance. Experimental approaches and data interpretation must take into account the certain but limited input of genetic factors into psychiatric disease, as well as unknown pathophysiology and trait identification.

No one waxes more eloquent or expert on behavioral genetics than Robert Plomin. In his essay "Beyond Nature versus Nurture," Plomin tracks the history of the swinging pendulum of nature versus nurture views, pronouncing the diminishing arc of this most unscientific debate. Quarrels over the supremacy of nature or nurture, in the abstract, lay intellectually defunct. We must acknowledge the input of both genes and environment (be it biological or psychosocial) and turn our attention to specific traits and illnesses. Surrender to an authentic scientific discussion leads to surprising and paradoxical results. By studying genetics, we have unearthed important information about the nature of environmental inputs. Also, the genetic nature of so-called environmental effects has become clear. Truth proves more astonishing and interesting than any embattled nature-versus-nurture fiction.

Irving Gottesman, the world's premier schizophrenia geneticist, lays out in his whimsically entitled essay the facts on schizophrenia inheritance. Many studies of various designs point to the role of genes in this most severe of mental illnesses. Existing genetic data also circumscribe the role of inherited factors in schizophrenia. Gottesman does more than posit the facts of schizophrenia genetics; he interpolates them into the realm of other theories about the origins of this disease. In an imaginary debate among a geneticist, virologist, and development scientist, the reader gains an appreciation of the many promising avenues of schizophrenia research and how these data may dovetail and overlap.

The gurus of mood disorder genetics, Ming Tsuang and Stephen Faraone, offer a detailed description of our current knowledge of the genetic input to major depression and bipolar disorder. A large volume of data undeniably point to the role of genes in these mood disorders. The complexity of mood disorders and their genetic underpinnings are also revealed. Mood disorders range in severity and symptom profiles; genetic mechanisms are likely to be equally complex. While a single gene may produce at least a subset of these conditions, more complicated arrangements likely contribute to mood disorders as well. Only a precise knowledge of the basic genetic data, laid out in this chapter, offers a clear vision of how to proceed and understand this research.

Mental illnesses affect the brain, the organ producing much of what is special and marvelous about human beings. How mental illnesses affect the brain and their relation to other mental functions is not clear, however. Kay Jamison, an accomplished researcher and author, embarks on a scientific consideration of the relationship between manic-depression and creativity. Scores of data point to a link between these two traits. While the nature of this association is not clear, the implications for the clinical psychiatric genetics may be profound. If prenatal testing and screening are applied to manic-depression on the finding of a major gene (a typical result of gene finds), we as a society may face the possibility of a depleted genetic substrate for creative work. Jamison harkens us to consider this potentiality.

The implications of psychiatric genetics are drawn out further by the eloquent and brave essay of Mary Ann Beall, a mental health consumer and family member of an individual with a serious mental illness. Genetic research and data can only be ethically and realistically brought forth by involving consumers and family members. They bring a reality to the discussion otherwise unseen. Beall tells of how genetics has resonated in her own path to understanding the illness from which she suffers. She also warns that a woefully inadequate service system is a poor, indeed impossible, foundation for the development of effective and humane clinical genetic services.

My own essay follows suit. In it, I discuss the many social domains relevant to psychiatric genetics and hold as preeminent the families and consumers in this debate. In the first instance, people with mental illnesses and their family members are necessary actors in research. Attention to their informed and ethical involvement stands as crucial. Second, people with mental illnesses and their family members will be the consumers of clinical genetic services. Indeed, they already clamor for such information. While the fairly well-developed principles of genetic counseling can be adapted to this purpose, little attention has been paid to this unmet need. Finally, I describe how the whole issue of psychiatric genetics plays out in a social milieu muddied by ignorance, stigma, and discrimination. As family members and consumers look to scientific data to free them from this terrible pit, they also must be clear as to the potential dangers that may lurk there. Psychiatric genetics, in this regard, is a double-edged sword.

The last essay, by the prolific and astute policy analyst Robert Mullan Cook-Deegan, grounds the concerns described above in the machinery of the federal government. The federal government has promulgated the major protections that exist for individuals participating in biomedical research. Cook-Deegan retells the fits and starts characterizing the development of these federal policies and highlights the missing pieces that make people with severe mental illnesses vulnerable.

These essays tell of a complicated yet promising scientific saga in the field of psychiatric genetics. Their message is clear: Further rigorous study is needed as is serious attention to the implications of science for people with mental illnesses, their family members, and our society at large.

CHAPTER 2

Evolution and Revolution in Psychiatric Genetics

CHARLES A. KAUFMANN, JANET E. JOHNSON, and
HERBERT PARDES

INTRODUCTION

Revolutionary advances in human genetics are having profound effects on
the theory and practice of medicine, and as genetic knowledge increases,
it is to be expected that its influence will only grow. Psychiatry is no
exception: clinical, molecular, and statistical genetic strategies promise to
reveal much about the etiology, pathogenesis, and treatment of mental
illness. In the foreseeable future, we hope to discover how the disposition
to mental illness is transmitted, the biological nature of the inherited factors,
and the ways in which these genetic factors interact with environmental determinants.

Psychiatric genetics encompasses both the genetics of psychiatric disease, such as alcoholism, bipolar disorder, dementia, and schizophrenia,
and the genetics of psychological capacities, traits, behaviors, and their
variations. While there is considerable interest in determining the genetics
and heritability of capacities like personality, or of consummatory, aggres-
sive, and sexual behaviors, these are beyond the scope of this chapter. Our
purpose here is to describe the role of contemporary genetics in understand-

CHARLES A. KAUFMANN, JANET E. JOHNSON, and HERBERT PARDES • Department of
Psychiatry, Columbia University, College of Physicians & Surgeons, New York, New York
10032.
Genetics and Mental Illness: Evolving Issues for Research and Society, edited by Laura Lee
Hall. Plenum Press, New York, 1996.

ing mental illness *per se.* We shall discuss the triumphs of positional cloning—the capacity to identify disease genes by virtue of their physical location within the genome—in elucidating the causes of genetically simple and
complex disorders. Next, we shall discuss the tribulations that this approach
has faced when applied to psychiatric disease. We shall attempt to place
these difficulties in a historical and philosophical context and to clarify
what makes genetically complex disorders so complex. We shall review
evolving approaches to simplifying these complexities, drawing on strategies
from clinical, molecular, and statistical genetics. Finally, we shall briefly
consider the implications of these developments for psychiatric nosology,
etiology, prevention, and treatment and speculate on their ethical, legal,
and social impact.

THE TRIUMPHS OF POSITIONAL CLONING

The recent identification of the gene underlying cystic fibrosis (CF), an
autosomal recessive disease, illustrates the profound capabilities of modern
genetics to elucidate the causes of human suffering. In unraveling this
enigmatic illness, the powerful techniques of molecular biology were used
to (1) determine the chromosomal location of the disease gene, (2) isolate
the gene itself, (3) identify the disease-causing mutation, and (4) produce
the abnormal protein product of the disease gene. Moreover, these findings
helped in clarifying the pathophysiological events leading to the initiation
and development of the disease, and facilitating the development of treatments directed at the fundamental biological defect in the disorder.

Using these techniques the causative gene for CF was localized to
a 1.5-million-base-pair (Mbp) interval of chromosome 7 (7q22.37–q23.1)
through linkage analysis in 1989. Subsequently, a collaborative effort identified a plausible candidate messenger RNA (mRNA) through additional
molecular techniques known as chromosome walking and chromosome
jumping. The 250,000-base-pair (bp) disease gene was isolated and was
found to encode a 6500-bp mRNA and a 1480-amino-acid protein. A 3-bp
deletion in a certain segment, exon 10, of the disease gene resulted in the
loss of a single amino acid, phenylalanine, in 70% of affected individuals.
This mutation (known as Δ F508) was never found in chromosomes from
normal individuals. The Δ F508 mutation has been associated with classic,
severe CF, with pancreatic insufficiency and meconium ileus.

Additional mutations of the same gene (currently numbering over 170)
have been identified and are associated with a variety of phenotypes, the
most mild of which constitute infertility in males in the absence of either
pulmonary or gastrointestinal symptoms. The product of the CF gene—cystic fibrosis transmembrane conductance regulator (CFTR)—was found to

be a member of a protein family involved in active transport across cell membranes, the traffic adenosine trisphosphatases. While all of the functions of CFTR remain to be elucidated, it appears to function as a chloride ion channel. Gene transfer of full-length, normal CFTR into CF epithelial cells corrects their chloride channel defect.

Additional *in vitro* analyses through transfection of the gene into a variety of cell types as well as expression in cell-free membrane patches have done much to clarify the role of CFTR as a chloride channel in the cell membrane, as a source of acidification of intracellular organelles, and as a protein affecting cyclic AMP-mediated endocytosis and exocytosis in both health and disease. In addition, Δ F508 CFTR has been introduced into mice to produce transgenic animals that mimic human CF pathology.

Finally, understanding of the basic pathophysiology of CF has directed the search for more effective treatments, ranging from efforts to activate the mutant forms of CFTR by increasing cytoplasmic cyclic AMP, to efforts to transfer a normal version of CFTR to appropriate target cells in the lungs through novel viral vectors, liposomes, or DNA–protein complexes (Collins, 1992).

Initially, these successes were achieved with genetically simple disorders, relatively rare illnesses demonstrating clear Mendelian modes of inheritance, e.g., CF (as noted, an autosomal recessive disorder), neurofibromatosis, type I (NF1) (an autosomal dominant disorder caused by a tumor-suppressor gene, neurofibromin, located near the centromere of chromosome 17 at 17q11.2) (Wallace *et al.,* 1990), and Duchenne muscular dystrophy (DMD) [an X-linked recessive disorder caused by a mutation in a gargantuan gene, dystrophin, spanning over 2,000,000 bp at Xp21.2, and coding for a protein involved in triadic junctions in skeletal muscle (Hoffman, Brown & Kunkel, 1987)] (Table 1). Not infrequently, success was facilitated by certain fortuitous clues, such as identifiable cytogenetic anomalies in affected individuals (as in NF1 and DMD), identifiable trinucleotide repeat expansions (as in Huntington's disease and dentatorubral pallidoluysian atrophy), or compelling candidate genes (as with fibrillin in Marfan syndrome) (Jorde, 1995).

More recently, major genes have been localized or identified for a number of genetically complex disorders, relatively common illnesses for which inheritance patterns are more obscure and in which genetic and environmental influences are felt to interact (Lander & Schork, 1994). For example, major genes for Hirschsprung disease, or aganglionic megacolon, long considered a clear example of polygenic inheritance (i.e., inheritance reflecting the consequence of innumerable, and thus undetectable, genes of small effect) (Passarge, 1993), have been mapped to chromosome 10q (dominant-acting) (Lyonnet *et al.,* 1993; Romeo *et al.,* 1994) and 13q (reces-

Table 1
Triumphs of Positional Cloning

Disorder	Inheritance	Major locus	Disease gene
Cystic fibrosis	Recessive	7q22–23	*CFTR*
Neurofibromatosis, type I	Dominant	17q11	*neurofibromin*
Duchenne muscular dystrophy	X-linked	Xp21	*dystrophin*
Hirschsprung disease	Complex	10q11	*RET proto-oncogene*
		13q22	—
Breast cancer	Complex	13q12–13	—
		17q21	*BRCA1*
Diabetes mellitus, type I	Complex	6p21	*MHC*
		11p15	*insulin*
Diabetes mellitus, type II	Complex	17q25	*glucagon receptor*

sive-acting) (Puffenberger *et al.*, 1994). Similarly, important genes contributing to familial breast cancer (BRCA1, BRCA2) (Miki *et al.*, 1994; Wooster *et al.*, 1994), type I (insulin-dependent) diabetes mellitus (IDDM) (HLA, insulin) (Davies *et al.*, 1994; Bennett *et al.*, 1995), and type II (non-insulin-dependent) diabetes mellitus (glucagon receptor) (Hager *et al.*, 1995), disorders with significant impact on public health, also have been identified (Table 1).

THE TRIBULATIONS OF PSYCHIATRIC GENETICS

Unfortunately, success in the application of positional cloning strategies to the study of other genetically complex illnesses, notably the psychiatric disorders, has been less predictable (Table 2). This has not been for lack of effort, however. Potential clues to disease pathogenesis have been exploited: the identification of a balanced trisomy of chromosome 5q11.2–13.3 in a Chinese-Canadian pedigree segregating schizophrenia (Bassett *et al.*, 1988), rapidly led to reports for (Sherrington *et al.*, 1988) and against (Kennedy *et al.*, 1988) linkage to this region. Several authors have argued for genetic anticipation, the phenomenological counterpart of trinucleotide repeat expansion, in both bipolar disorder (McInnis *et al.*, 1993) and schizophrenia (Bassett & Honer, 1994), and other authors have directly sought

Table 2
Tribulations of Psychiatric Genetics

Disorder	Major locus/allele	Replication[a]
Alcoholism	D_2 receptor A1 (11q)	−
Alzheimer disease	Apolipoprotein E ε4 (19q)	+
	14q24	+
	21q11–21	+
Bipolar disorder	11p15	−
	18cen	+/−
	21	?
	Xq27–28	−
Schizophrenia	D_3 receptor (3q)[b]	−
	5q11–13	−
	6p21–22	+
	22q12–13	+/−

[a] +, replicated; −, unreplicated; +/−, equivocal; ?, unavailable.
[b] Homozygosity.

such expansions (J. Kennedy and C. Ross, personal communications), yet reports of anticipation are potentially confounded by inescapable ascertainment biases (S. Hodge, personal communication). There have been a number of candidate gene studies, notably of the dopamine (D_2, D_3) receptor genes in alcoholism (Blum & Noble, 1990) and schizophrenia (Crocq et al., 1992), studies that have not withstood replication (Gelernter, Goldman, & Risch, 1993; Coon et al., 1993). Similarly, even "findings" made without the benefit of (potentially misleading) clues have not survived the test of time: initial evidence for major gene loci underlying bipolar disorder on chromosomes 11 (Egeland, Gerhard, & Pauls, 1987) and X (Baron et al., 1987) has subsequently received diminished support in the very same datasets in which they appeared (Kelsoe et al., 1989; Baron et al., 1993).

All news arising from gene scans for psychiatric disorders is not bad, however. For example, major gene loci either causing or affecting the course of at least some cases of Alzheimer disease have been identified on chromosomes 14 (Schellenberg et al., 1992; St George-Hyslop et al., 1992), 19 (apolipoprotein E e4 allele) (Corder et al., 1993), and 21 (amyloid precursor protein (Goate et al., 1991). There are promising loci for bipolar disorder on chromosomes 18 (Berrettini, Ferraro, Goldin, et al., 1994) and 21 (Straub et al., 1994), and promising loci for schizophrenia on chromosomes 6 (K. Kendler & R. Straub, personal communication) and 22 (Pulver et al., 1994).

EVOLUTION AND REVOLUTION IN CONTEMPORARY GENETICS

Despite these encouraging signs, progress in the search for psychiatric susceptibility loci has been slow, and not always steady. Impediments to positional cloning may best be understood by placing the *revolutionary* advances in human genetics into an *evolutionary* (i.e., historical and philosophical) context. This historical and philosophical context, in turn, may best be understood by making reference to Thomas Kuhn's view of scientific progress, as enunciated in his landmark essay, *The Structure of Scientific Revolutions* (1970). Kuhn contended that the usual scientific undertaking, which he called "normal science," was rarely concerned with identifying phenomenal or conceptual novelties. Rather, governed by an implicit "paradigm" or world view, it focused on articulating derivative theories, determining significant facts, and, ultimately, matching these facts and theories; that is, it was mostly concerned with solving puzzles. Despite this epistemological conservatism, scientific inquiry inevitably unearthed "anomalies," phenomena that withstood explanation by the prevailing paradigm. Anomalies begot scientific crises, and crises begot (revolutionary) shifts in the underlying paradigm.

Viewed in this light, contemporary concepts of molecular pathogenesis may be seen to derive from distinct theories of etiology, pathophysiology, and nosology, theories that are interrelated by reference to common world views, and that have undergone gradual modifications punctuated by abrupt paradigm shifts. The underlying paradigms, arbitrarily designated the "continual," the "elemental," and the "dialectical," and their relationships to etiology, pathophysiology, and nosology are enumerated in Table 3.

References to the transmission of familial traits can be traced back to the beginnings of recorded history. Ancient civilizations utilized basic genetic principles in breeding animals and plants in an effort to improve their physical characteristics. The Greeks proposed the theory of *pangenesis,* which stated that traits were inherited through and blended in the blood, a principle that has endured for nearly 2000 years and has found modern

Table 3
Shifting Genetic Paradigms

Paradigm	Etiology	Pathophysiology	Nosology	Example
Continual	Polygenic	Humoral	Syndromal	Pyloric stenosis
Elemental	Monogenic	Molecular	Mutational	Cystic fibrosis
Dialectical	Multifactorial	Interactive	Susceptibility	Diabetes mellitus

expression in Galtonian notions of quantitative, polygenic inheritance. Similarly, the *Corpus Hippocraticum* (ca. 400 B.C.) identified imbalances in the four bodily humors as instrumental to the development of disease. Thomas Sydenham (1624–1689), the "English Hippocrates," likewise implicated quantitative disturbances in bodily fluids (along with climate and diet) in the development of pathological syndromes, as well as defining such syndromes as illnesses sharing signs and outcome. These theories of etiology, pathophysiology, and nosology all rely on the underlying concept of a continuum of normal and abnormal transmissible traits: consequently, we have designated the (implicit) paradigm on which they are based as the "continual" paradigm. Pyloric stenosis exemplifies a "continual" genetic disorder: risk to affected individuals is well predicted by a quantitative threshold model with risk to offspring lying midway between the parental and population means, increasing with greater family burden of illness, and precipitously decreasing with decreasing degree of relationship (Carter, 1964).

The "continual" paradigm was eventually superseded by the atomistic or "elemental" paradigm. Although the origins of the latter paradigm also can be traced to the Greeks [Democritus of Abdera (ca. 500 B.C.)], it was not until the 17th century that it came to govern scientific and medical thought. Over the ensuing centuries, the quest for the fundamental building blocks of health and disease has led investigators to successively examine the anatomic [William Harvey (1578–1657)], cellular [Rudolf Virchow (1821–1902)], and molecular [Archibald Garrod (1902)] levels of biology. The "elemental" paradigm has led to the exploratory juggernaut of contemporary molecular biology, "normal science" at its best. The evolution of this paradigm is well known: in 1865, Gregor Mendel applied scientific methodology to the question of hereditary and proposed his now-famous laws. His work went largely unnoticed until the early 1900s, when it was rediscovered by European biologists. Thomas Hunt Morgan and his colleagues at Columbia University produced the first genetic map in the first decade of the 20th century using the fruit fly. In 1911, the first human gene, that for color blindness, was correctly assigned to a particular chromosome. In 1953, Watson and Crick elucidated the double-helical structure of DNA. Hybrid and chemical staining techniques were discovered in the 1960s, thus facilitating genetic mapping. By the mid-1970s, several genes had been assigned to the X chromosome as well as to some of the autosomes, through functional cloning, the technique of isolating a gene through its associated protein. Restriction fragment length polymorphisms (RFLPs) were widely used beginning in the late 1970s and enabled the successful localization of the gene for Huntington disease in 1983. Since then, molecular genetic techniques have expanded at a remarkable pace, propelled in part by the discovery of the polymerase chain reaction (PCR) and microsatellite (short tandem repeat) polymorphisms, and have made the prospect of mapping the 50,000–100,000 genes that comprise the human genome a realistic goal. This goal will undoubtedly be achieved through the efforts of the Human Genome Project (HGP), an international collaborative research initiative organized to produce detailed genetic and physical maps of each of the 24 human chromosomes and to determine the sequence of the 3 billion nucleotides that make up human DNA. A 1-centimorgan (cM) (a genetic distance approximately equal to 1 Mbp) genetic map has already been realized [Cooperative Human Linkage Center (CHLC)/Centre D'Etude Polymorphisme Humain (CEPH), 1994]. The HGP is expected to be completed by the year 2000, at an estimated cost of $3 billion.

The "elemental" paradigm has inspired (one might even say, dictated) the search for single gene mutations underlying illness. One need only peruse the more than 3000 ostensibly single gene disorders described in *Mendelian Inheritance in Man* (McKusick, 1992) to see how pervasive this paradigm has become. CF typifies the "elemental" aphorism: one mutation/ one disease, with clear implications for nosology. Thus, the CFTR Δ F508 mutation has come to be associated with CF with pancreatic insufficiency (CF-PI), a disorder with clear symptomatology, pathophysiology, and course of illness (early onset, poor prognosis), while those CF patients lacking the Δ F508 mutation perforce have a different disease, CF with pancreatic sufficiency (CF-PS).

We would contend that contemporary genetics is in the throes of a shift in world view, from the exclusive "elemental" to a more inclusive, "dialectical," paradigm. No longer do monogenic theories of etiology suffice to explain the complex interplay of multiple genetic and environmental risk factors. Moreover, genes do not simply cause disease: they confer susceptibility. Under the "dialectical" paradigm, specific gene mutations are no longer sufficient, and may not even be necessary, to cause a specific disorder. As articulated by Kendler and Eaves (1986), three fundamental models account for the joint effect of genes and environment on liability to illness (within the "dialectical" paradigm).

The first model, additive genetic and environmental effects, hypothesizes that liability to illness results from the simple addition of the genetic and environmental contributions. The second model, genetic control of sensitivity to the environment, proposes that genes control the degree to which an individual is sensitive to either risk-increasing or risk-reducing aspects of the environment. The third model, genetic control of exposure to the environment, postulates that a genotype's influence on the liability to illness is to alter the probability of exposure to a predisposing environment. Within the "dialectical" paradigm, notions of interactive etiology find their counterpart in notions of interactive pathophysiology. This is well illustrated by contemporary neurobiological theories of synaptic plasticity and learning, wherein the efficiency of genetically programmed synaptic connections is modified by exposure to environmental stimuli (E. Kandel, personal communication).

Finally, as pyloric stenosis typifies the "continual" paradigm, and CF exemplifies the "elemental" paradigm, IDDM epitomizes the "dialectical" paradigm. IDDM is characterized by autoimmune destruction of the insulin-producing β cells of the pancreatic islets of Langerhans. While variations at several genetic loci confer susceptibility to the illness (Davies *et al.,* 1994), almost half of the genetic risk is determined by polymorphisms within the peptide-binding sites of the class II major histocompatibility complex (MHC, HLA) molecules HLA-DQ and HLA-DR located on chromosome 6p21 (IDDM1). Class II MHC molecules, expressed at the surface of antigen-presenting cells (APCs), are responsible for binding and presenting peptides, derived from the limited proteolysis of foreign proteins internalized by the APCs, to T cells. A compelling model of IDDM pathogenesis suggests that specific Class II MHC molecules orchestrate an immune response to the enterovirus, Coxsackie virus B (CoxB). Because of "molecular mimicry" (i.e., amino acid sequence homology) between the P2-C protein of CoxB and the enzyme, glutamic acid decarboxylase (GAD65), of β cells, this protective immune response causes unwanted "collateral damage" with the eventual pathologic destruction of β cells (Solimena & De Camilli, 1995). This role for GAD65 autoimmunity in the pathogenesis of IDDM is supported by studies in humans and mice [with the nonobese diabetes (NOD) mouse developing autoimmune diabetes and early appearing autoantibodies to GAD65]; in what follows, we shall have more to say about the importance of animal models in simplifying the complexities of complex disorders. As noted, loci other than MHC also confer susceptibility to IDDM. The second most important locus appears in the vicinity of the insulin gene itself (chromosome 11p15.5): it would appear that allelic variations in a minisatellite (VNTR) polymorphism upstream to the insulin coding region influence *in vivo* insulin mRNA transcription and, consequently, disease susceptibility (Bennett *et al.,* 1995).

With this historical and philosophical background in mind, those difficulties that have been encountered in the positional cloning of psychiatric disorders become more understandable. Complex disorders represent Kuhnian "anomalies" for the "elemental" paradigm. They are not easily explained by single Mendelian genes.

COMPLEXITIES OF COMPLEX DISORDERS

On the other hand, the "dialectical" paradigm provides for many of the complexities that characterize complex disorders. These are listed in Table 4, along with clinical examples drawn from the study of IDDM and one psychiatric disorder, schizophrenia.

As can be seen from Table 4, IDDM and schizophrenia share many characteristics. Neither demonstrates a clear Mendelian mode of inheritance, and dominant, recessive, additive (i.e., intermediate gene dosage), and oligogenic (i.e., multilocus) forms have been proposed for both. The various transmitted forms may reflect various genetic, environmental, and interactive etiologies all resulting in a common phenotype (see Hyde, Ziegler, & Weinberger, 1992). As regards IDDM, genetic heterogeneity for glucose intolerance also has been well documented in rodent models

Table 4
Complexities of Complex Disorders

Complexity	Diabetes (IDDM)	Schizophrenia
Unknown mode of inheritance	Dominant, recessive, additive, oligogenic all proposed	Dominant, recessive, additive, oligogenic all proposed
Etiologic heterogeneity	Over 60 rare genetic disorders with glucose intolerance; heterogeneity in rodent models	A variety of neuropsychiatric disorders (e.g., metachromatic leukodystrophy) with psychosis
Variable expression	Variations in age of onset, clinical presentation (ketosis versus vascular complications), insulin autoantibodies, viral antibodies	Variations in age of onset, clinical presentation (psychosis, affective symptoms), neuronal autoantibodies, viral antibodies
Incomplete penetrance	MZ twin concordance 36%	MZ twin concordance 59%
Epistasis	*IDDM1-5,7;* multiple susceptibility loci in the NOD mouse	Presumed, based on optimal model-fitting with 3-locus model
Loci of small effect	*IDDM3* (15q), 4 (11q), 5 (6q), 7 (2q)	Presumed
Multifactorial etiology	HLA, insulin, coxsackie virus	Possibly, HLA, influenza virus
Diagnostic instability	Present	Present

(e.g., the NOD mouse, the BB rat). That is, there is no one-to-one correspondence between genotype and phenotype. This correspondence breaks down in other ways. In both disorders, presumably single genetic forms result in a panoply of phenotypic expressions. Animal models of diabetes suggest that the genetic background of the individual (including its gender) may influence this expression (Leiter, Coleman, & Hummel, 1981). Not all monozygotic (MZ) twins are concordant for either IDDM or schizophrenia (i.e., both disorders demonstrate incomplete penetrance), suggesting that what is inherited in each disorder is not disease, but disease susceptibility, susceptibility that must interact with other (presumably environmental or stochastic) factors to produce clinical symptoms. As noted previously, at least two loci of major effect (HLA, insulin) and four loci of minor effect have been implicated in human IDDM; similarly, up to five independent loci have been implicated in diabetes susceptibility in the NOD mouse (one of which is H-2, the murine counterpart of HLA) (Todd et al., 1991). While epistasis (gene interaction) has not been demonstrated for schizophrenia, optimal model-fitting to empirical recurrence risk data suggests that at least three loci may contribute to the disorder (Risch, 1990). Of course, the more loci that are implicated in the pathogenesis of a disorder, the smaller their individual effect on the disease phenotype. This has been demonstrated for the minor loci in both human and murine diabetes, and is presumed to pertain to schizophrenia. This is not surprising if one considers that many loci, significantly affecting a variety of quantitative traits in experimental organisms such as maize, contribute less than 5% of the variance of the final phenotype. Finally, as previously discussed, it would appear that a variety of genetically determined host factors (such as specific HLA alleles like DR4) interact with epigenetic environmental factors (like Coxsackie viruses) to produce IDDM. Conceivably, host genes and viruses could also interact to produce the schizophrenia phenotype. In this regard, it is interesting to note that (1) recent (provisionally replicated) evidence for a schizophrenia susceptibility locus at 6p21–22 implicates the HLA region contained therein, (2) prenatal influenza virus infection has long been suggested as an environmental risk factor in the development of schizophrenia, and (3) patients with schizophrenia bear many of the stigmata of autoimmune (possibly viral-mediated) injury, including CD56 T lymphocytes and autoantibodies against the 60-Kda heat shock protein.

The "dialectical" paradigm, allowing as it does for multifactorial etiology, interactive pathophysiology, and nosologic groupings based on disease susceptibility (rather than disease itself), readily accommodates these complexities of complex disorders.

SIMPLIFYING THE COMPLEXITIES OF COMPLEX DISORDERS: ADVANCES IN CLINICAL, MOLECULAR, AND STATISTICAL GENETICS

In the section that follows, we shall describe a number of advances in clinical, molecular, and statistical genetics that may facilitate the discovery of susceptibility loci underlying genetically complex diseases, of which psychiatric disorders are representative (Table 5).

Clinical Genetics

Recent advances in clinical genetics that may facilitate the study of psychiatric disorders include refinements in clinical populations and phenotypes for study along with increasing reliance on animal models of disease.

Many of the complexities of complex disorders such as etiologic heterogeneity and epistasis can be resolved by sheer numbers, and there has been an increasing reliance on large samples and clinical consortia to address this issue. Thus, the aforementioned genome-wide search for human type I diabetes susceptibility genes relied on almost 300 sibling pairs affected with the disorder (Davies *et al.*, 1994). Etiologic heterogeneity can also be resolved by studying populations in which genetic bottlenecks have occurred (i.e., in which a finite number of founders limit the number of disease genes entering a population). Geographically and/or ethnically isolated

Table 5
Simplifying the Complexities

Complexity	Clinical	Molecular	Statistical
Unknown mode of inheritance	+[a]		+
Etiologic heterogeneity	+		+
Variable expression			+
Incomplete penetrance	+		+
Epistasis	+	+	+
Loci of small effect		+	
Multifactorial etiology			
Diagnostic instability	+		

[a]Approach described in text to simplify the complexity shown.

populations have been employed in the study of a number of disorders, including bipolar affective disorder in the Old Order Amish (Egeland *et al.*, 1987) and diastrophic dysplasia in Finland (Hastbacka *et al.*, 1992). Such populations are also useful for particular statistical approaches, such as linkage disequilibrium mapping *(vide infra)*. The sensitivity of linkage results to diagnostic misspecification [e.g., "lifetime" diagnoses of depression may paradoxically change over the course of a lifetime (Rice *et al.*, 1987), obese NIDM patients may lose all clinical and chemical signs of the disorder if their weight returns to normal (Rotter, Vadheim, & Rimoin, 1992] may be avoided by examining both nuclear and extensive pedigrees (Pauls, 1993).

Genetic studies of psychiatric and other complex disorders have increasingly turned away from categorical, polychotomous definitions of illness, to quantitative measures of disease. Frequently, "endophenotypes," disease-associated physiological abnormalities demonstrating Mendelian inheritance and complete penetrance, are sought. Thus, subclinical phenotypes like psychometric deviation (Moldin *et al.*, 1990) and psychophysiological gating impairment (Waldo *et al.*, 1991) have been described in schizophrenia, while measurements of fasting and glucose-challenge-induced plasma glucose levels have been incorporated into diagnostic criteria for diabetes (National Diabetes Data Group, 1979).

In addition, animal models of human disease may have particular salience for the understanding of complex disorders. Consider the mouse. Hundreds of inbred and mutant strains exist, thousands of microsatellite markers have been mapped (59 genes have been positionally cloned), and proposed disease genes may be introduced via transgenesis, allowing Koch's central postulate, disease transmission, to be directly tested. The use of mice allows new genes to be identified through quantitative trait locus mapping [they have been instrumental in the discovery of genes contributing to two complex behavioral disorders, obesity and opiate preference (Zhang *et al.*, 1994; Berrettini, Ferraro, Alexander, *et al.*, 1994)], allow the physiological consequences of known genes to be assessed, and permit a detailed understanding of the roles of gene interaction and (polygenic) genetic "background" in gene expression. It is not surprising, therefore, that the 1990s has been designated the "decade of the mouse" (Paigen, 1995).

Molecular Genetics

Complementing these clinical approaches have been a number of molecular genetic developments, including approaches to rapid genome scanning for candidate genes, as well as for anonymous genomic segments shared between affected individuals or differing between affected and suitably matched unaffected individuals. These approaches promise to identify many, if not all, epistatic loci contributing to complex disorders, even if their contribution to overall phenotypic variation is most modest.

Thus, over 80,000 partially sequenced complementary DNAs (cDNAs) (clones that are complementary to endogenous mRNAs), also known as expressed sequence tags (ESTs), have been placed onto the physical map of the genome. While the sequences that are currently available often only partially represent full-length mRNAs and are to some degree redundant with one another, a major step toward a transcriptional map, i.e., a physical map of all 100,000 genes that are thought to comprise the human genome, has been achieved. Moreover, the profound implications for psychiatric genetics are apparent, if one considers that over half of these genes are exclusively expressed in brain (Adams *et al.*, 1992). Specific sets of these genes that are expressed in particular brain regions, or during particular neurodevelopment stages, implicated in the pathoetiology of specific disorders, (e.g., the hippocampus and second gestational trimester, respectively, in schizophrenia) may be directly cloned through the techniques of library normalization and subtractive hybridization (M.B. Soares, personal communication). Other potentially pathogenic sequences, such as expanded trinucleotide repeats which, to date, have been implicated in the development of nine neuropsychiatric disorders, may be directly isolated (J. Kennedy and C. Ross, personal communications). Once these complete sets or specific subsets of candidate genes are isolated, their roles in particular diseases may be rapidly evaluated through advances in linkage disequilibrium scanning (Pacek, Sajantila, & Syvanen, 1993; J. A. Knowles, personal communication) and mutation detection.

These "candidate" gene approaches depend on first "nominating" the candidate (either through specific associations with neuroanatomic regions, neurodevelopmental stages, or neuropathic changes like trinucleotide repeat expansion) and then having the candidate "run for office." Of course, ESTs represent the ideal participatory democracy, with *everyone* in the race. On the other hand, two additional extraordinary approaches being developed, genomic mismatch scanning (GMS) and representational difference analysis (RDA), promise to elect genes directly, bypassing the primaries and conventions. Both approaches may be especially useful in detecting multiple genes acting in concert to produce disease.

GMS is a molecular technique to isolate all regions of *identity* (by descent) between two individuals, based on the ability of these regions to form extensive mismatch-free heteroduplex DNA molecules (Nelson *et al.*, 1993). GMS is most powerful when used to compare the DNA of distantly related affected individuals, especially in pedigrees from isolated populations having undergone genetic "bottlenecks." Application of this technique should permit the identification of regions as small as 10 kb (the approximate size of individual genes) which contribute to disease expression. The technique has been demonstrated to work in yeast and experiments to extend it to humans are in progress (P. Brown, personal communication).

Conversely, RDA is a molecular technique for cloning the *difference* between two complex genomes (Lisitsyn *et al.*, 1993). In this method, restriction endonuclease fragments which differ in length between two individuals [so-called polymorphic amplifiable restriction endonuclease fragments (PARFs)] are selectively enriched by repetitive subtractive hybridization. PARFs, so generated, will be linked to the phenotypic trait that discriminates the two individuals. They are generated without knowledge of the chromosomal location(s) of the gene(s) controlling the trait; in fact, once generated, they can direct the search for such locations. Thus, in actuality, RDA represents neither functional *nor* positional cloning. The RDA approach has been successfully used to directly isolate polymorphic markers linked to phenotypic traits in congenic experimental organisms, those that are genetically identical except for a relatively small region surrounding a gene of interest (Lisitsyn *et al.*, 1994). In extending this approach to human diseases, significantly inbred populations may be particularly informative.

Statistical Genetics

Statistical genetics represents the third pillar of contemporary human genetics, and here, too, rapid advances promise to pave the way to the identification of psychiatric susceptibility genes. Statistical developments promise to facilitate phenotype definition, efficient and sensitive linkage analysis, and more powerful linkage disequilibrium analysis, thereby surmounting obstacles to positional cloning presented by unknown mode of inheritance, incomplete penetrance, and etiologic heterogeneity.

Multivariate approaches to phenotype definition (such as pedigree discriminant analysis) may allow integrated statistical phenotypes demonstrating Mendelian inheritance patterns, and thus possibly reflecting single gene effects, to be identified (Zlotnik, Elston, & Namboodiri, 1983). Conversely, other approaches, like phenometric analysis, may allow detection of differentiated phenotypic features resulting from individual genetic loci (George *et al.*, 1987). Multitiered approaches to linkage analysis [initially screening with widely spaced markers and maximizing sensitivity at the expense of specificity (Elston, 1994)] may permit more rapid genomic scanning, a boon for oligogenic disorders in which the serendipitous discovery of a single major locus may only be the beginning of the search for several susceptibility genes. Nonparametric approaches to linkage analysis [such as affected sib pair (Davies *et al.*, 1994) and affected pedigree member strategies (Weeks & Lange, 1993)] may be robust in the face of model misspecification (again a plus for disorders in which genetic models are unknown), while other approaches (such as bivariate analyses combining categorical disease definitions with quantitative phenotype measures) (S.O. Moldin, personal communication) may increase the power to detect loci in the face of etiologic heterogeneity. The ability of nonallelic genetic heterogeneity to weaken linkage analyses can be offset by statistical approaches that allow for such heterogeneity (MacLean *et al.*, 1992). Given the possibility of undetected heterogeneity, however, greater caution may need to be adopted in reporting that linkage has been excluded from particular chromosomal regions (Pakstis *et al.*, 1991).

Despite these developments, the various complexities of complex disorders (e.g., uncertain genetic model, oligogenic inheritance) conspire to hinder linkage replication (Suarez, Hampe, & van Eerdewegh, 1994) and to render the exact genetic location of linked loci uncertain (L. Sandkuijl, personal communication), even if these loci can be detected. Thus, linkage analysis for a psychiatric disorder may localize a susceptibility locus to a region spanning 20–30 cM, far beyond the 1- to 2-cM capabilities of current physical mapping and gene isolation strategies. Even this obstacle, however, may be circumvented through developments in linkage disequilibrium or shared segment scanning, an alternative approach to linkage analysis in which strings of alleles (haplotypes) surrounding disease loci will be shared among affected individuals. These strategies may be especially effective in "bottleneck" populations derived from a small number of progenitors (Houwen *et al.*, 1995; de la Chapelle, 1993).

In summary, rapid advances on all three fronts bode well for the eventual identification of many, if not all, genes that significantly contribute to heritable psychiatric disorders. The detection, localization, identification, and characterization of these genes will undoubtedly provide an important focus for basic and clinical neurosciences for years to come. In the next, concluding section, we shall speculate on the developments those years may bring.

FUTURE DIRECTIONS

The identification of major susceptibility genes for Alzheimer disease, alcoholism, bipolar disorder, schizophrenia, and other psychiatric disorders can be expected to result in significant changes in our concepts of psychiatric nosology, etiology, and therapeutics.

Nosology

Traditionally, nosologists have been divided into two camps: "splitters" and "lumpers." Advances in psychiatric genetics may provide insights to satisfy both camps. "Splitters" will be gratified to see that disorders, like Alzheimer disease, once thought to represent single diseases, may reflect a number of disorders sharing a final common path to neurodegeneration but differing in important clinical features like age of onset. As we have seen, this has been the case with cystic fibrosis. "Lumpers" will be happy to see that psychopathology, like depression and anxiety, once thought to represent separate disorders, may reflect a common genetic base with alternative phenotypic expressions (Kendler *et al.*, 1987). Similarly, other symptomatic features, like psychosis, may ultimately prove to reflect major gene effects that cut across current nosologic boundaries (such as the one that currently separates bipolar disorder and schizophrenia) (Tsuang & Lyons, 1989).

Etiology

The identification of major genes may yield unexpected dividends, namely, clearer specification of polygenic and nongenetic (or better, epigenetic/environmental) factors that influence disease penetrance and expression. Epigenetic influences might extend from the womb to the tomb, and range from pre-, peri-, and postnatal biological insults to shared intrafamilial conflict (like parental divorce or death) to nonshared, unique traumas (mediated by birth order, temperament, between-sib strife, etc.) (Reiss, Plomin, & Hetherington, 1991). Clearly, environmental influences need not be exclusively permissive; to the extent that protective influences can be identified, nongenetic approaches to the prevention and treatment of ostensibly genetic disorders may be developed.

Prevention and Treatment

In fact, there are many stages in the development of multifactorial psychiatric disorders that may be amenable to therapeutic intervention: consequently, such intervention may be viewed as achieving primary, secondary, or tertiary prevention. Regarding primary prevention, genetic discoveries may permit more informed genetic counseling, which historically has had to rely on unsatisfactory empirical risk data. This may allow realistic reproductive options to be exercised, especially in families heavily burdened by illness. Primary prevention may also involve gene therapy. This, in turn, may be direct (i.e., genetic engineering of somatic or germline cells) or indirect (as in the previously described efforts to pharmacologically compensate for mutations in CF by increasing airway epithelial cell cytoplasmic cyclic AMP, or in efforts to compensate for β-hemoglobin deficiencies in thalassemia by inducing the atavistic expression of immature, but serviceable, embryonic ε-hemoglobin). Furthermore, while the anatomically complex and remote central nervous system was once thought to be inaccessible to direct gene therapy, the development of novel neurotropic viral vectors and engrafted *(ex vivo)* genetically transformed mature cells or immature but pleuripotential neural progenitor cells (cells that assume the phenotypic characteristics of cell types common to the brain region to which they are grafted) all suggest that direct gene therapy for neuropsychiatric disorders may soon be a matter of science fact, not of science fiction.

Secondary prevention may be achieved *prenatally,* in disorders like schizophrenia thought to develop in response to adverse *in utero* experiences. Pregnancies of fetuses at special genetic risk might be monitored more closely, and shielded from identified epigenetic risks factors like prenatal micronutrient deficiencies or viral exposures. Tertiary prevention might be achieved *postnatally* in schizophrenia and other disorders, to the extent that high-risk presymptomatic individuals could be reliably identified and acute illness forestalled. Such interventions might be especially important, if, as has been proposed, florid symptoms of both bipolar disorder and schizophrenia are pathogenic in their own right (e.g., through kindling or free-radical-induced neurotoxicity).

Social Implications

The identification of major genes conferring vulnerability to psychiatric disorders may also have important social implications, in such areas as ethics, the law, discrimination, and genetic counseling. The HGP has established an Ethical, Legal, and Social Implications (ELSI) program in response to concerns over these implications.

Ethical implications of the new medical genetics relate to such issues as confidentiality and privacy, equity, and extending the role of patient beyond the individual initially seeking treatment to other family members. Another concern is one that has already arisen with Huntington disease, namely, the additional risk that attends the notification of genetic risk status, especially for serious neuropsychiatric disorders for which a diagnosis can be made but no treatment provided.

Psychiatric genetics has all of the ethical concerns of medical genetics, as well as additional concerns. By the very nature of their illnesses, patients with psychiatric disorders often have impaired judgment and limited insight, deficits that result in decreased autonomy, increased paternalism, and necessarily greater reliance on institutional ethical safeguards.

In relation to the law, we can anticipate that the ability to identify individuals at genetic risk for psychiatric disorders, along with ambiguity regarding the threshold between genetic susceptibility and genetic affliction, will have important implications for the concept of diminished capacity and culpability.

Psychiatric disorders present all of the risks of genetic discrimination inherent in other medical disorders, along with additional risks. The risk of genetic discrimination, defined by Goston (1991) as "the denial of rights, privileges, or opportunities on the basis of information obtained from genetically-based diagnostic and prognostic tests," is real and exists in several arenas, including insurance coverage, employment, and social stigma. This is particularly true in the case of mental illnesses for which discrimination and stigma are already realities. For example, mental health insurance benefits are invariably less than those for other medical conditions.

Stigma has oppressed the mentally ill for over 500 years (Foucault, 1965). While we can hope that psychiatric disorders, as complex illnesses, will be recognized as worthy of the same concern, consideration, and compassion as the other complex illnesses we have described, and while we can hope that the revolutionary advances in genetic understanding we have heralded will be accompanied by revolutionary changes in social attitudes, past history would suggest otherwise. Over the past century, psychiatric genetics has all too often been a willing instrument of stigma, frequently in the name of eugenics. Eugenics, derived from the Greek words *eu,* meaning "well," and *genos,* meaning "born," refers to the concept of improving a race by the bearing of healthy offspring (Garver & Garver, 1991). Both positive and negative eugenics have been proposed, with the former referring to a systematic effort to maximize the transmission of genes that are considered desirable, and the latter referring to a systematic effort to minimize the transmission of genes that are considered deleterious. The eugenics movement within Nazi Germany has been the subject of universal outrage. The primary targets of this movement were the so-called "feeble-minded" and persons with psychiatric illnesses. Many of these individuals were involuntarily sterilized; many others were murdered. Less well known, but no less worrisome, has been the eugenics movement within the United States during the first half of this century. The possibility of a resurgence of eugenic policies cannot be ignored.

Psychiatrists are especially well equipped, by nature of their training, to help people with the feelings, concerns, and issues raised by hereditary illnesses, be they psychiatric or otherwise (Pardes *et al.,* 1989). The emotional impact of genetic disease is great. It is accompanied by serious concerns regarding whom to test, when to offer testing, and how to interpret results to patients. These concerns are laden with ethical as well as psychotherapeutic issues. The traditional role of genetic counseling has been to impart information concerning the nature of the illness, recurrence risks, anticipated burden of care, and reproductive options in a nondirective way. Often, counseling has been conducted by a team of genetic specialists including genetically trained clinicians and genetic counselors. As genetic knowledge continues to expand, the need for genetic counseling services will dramatically increase; the concern has been voiced that sufficient genetic counseling services may not be available to meet this increased demand. Whatever form psychiatric genetic counseling takes, it will be essential that it maintains its nondirective approach, as well as a regard for such important ethical principles as autonomy, confidentiality, privacy, informed consent, and voluntariness.

CONCLUSION

Throughout this chapter we have emphasized the remarkable transformation that contemporary genetics has brought to all of medicine, including psychiatry. Technological advances, along with a fundamental change in the ways we view disease, have elucidated the etiology and pathophysiology of a number of genetically simple, Mendelian disorders. Inspired by this success, geneticists now have turned their attention to more common, costly, and complex conditions. Here, too, positional cloning has revealed important genetic determinants of illnesses ranging from breast cancer to diabetes to hypertension. Psychiatric illnesses are likely to be no more complex, and we can anticipate that major genes contributing to alcoholism, Alzheimer disease, bipolar disorder, schizophrenia, and a host of other ailments will soon be in hand. We can also anticipate that these genetic discoveries will provide important insights into the influence of nongenetic factors on psychiatric disease expression, into the basic pathophysiology of brain disruption, and into novel therapeutic interventions. Undoubtedly, expanding knowledge will bring with it expanded responsibilities. Nonetheless, we stand on the threshold of a new and exciting era of discovery, one that seems certain to revolutionize the ways in which we view our patients, their illnesses, and the tools at our disposal to offer them relief.

ACKNOWLEDGMENTS

The authors wish to thank Ms. Kelly George for help in the preparation of the manuscript. This work was supported in part by grant K02 MH00682 from the National Institutes of Health.

REFERENCES

Adams, M. D., Dubnick, M., Kerlavage, A. R., et al. (1992). Sequence identification of 2,375 human brain genes. Nature, 355, 632–634.
Baron, M., Risch, N., Hamburger, R., et al. (1987). Genetic linkage between X chromosome markers and bipolar affective illness. Nature, 326, 289–292.
Baron, M., Freimer, N., Risch, N., et al. (1993). Diminished support for linkage between manic depressive illness and x-chromosome markers in three Israeli pedigrees. Nature Genetics, 3, 49–55.
Bassett, A. S., & Honer, W. G. (1994). Evidence for anticipation in schizophrenia. American Journal of Human Genetics, 54, 864–870.
Bassett, A. S., McGillivray, B. C., Jones, B., & Pantzar, J. T. (1988). Partial trisomy chromosome 5 cosegregating with schizophrenia. Lancet, I, 799–801.
Bennett, S. T., Lucassen, A. M., Gough, S. C. L., et al. (1994). Susceptibility to human type 1 diabetes at IDDM2 is determined by tandem repeat variation at the insulin gene minisatellite locus. Nature Genetics, 9, 284–291.
Berrettini, W. H., Ferraro, T. N., Alexander, R. C., et al. (1994). Quantitative trait loci mapping of three loci controlling morphine preference using inbred mouse strains. Nature Genetics, 7, 54–58.
Berrettini, W. H., Ferraro, T. N., Goldin, L. R., et al. (1994). Chromosome 18 DNA markers and manic-depressive illness: Evidence for a susceptibility gene. Proceedings of the National Academy of Sciences (USA), 91, 5918–5921.
Blum, K., & Noble, E. (1990). Allelic association of human dopamine D_2 receptor gene in alcoholism. Journal of the American Medical Association, 18, 2055–2060.
Carter, C. O. (1964). The genetics of common malformations. In M. Fishbein (Ed.), Congenital malformations: Papers and discussions presented at the Second International Conference on Congenital Malformations (pp. 306–313). New York: International Medical Congress.
Collins, F. S. (1992). Cystic fibrosis: Molecular biology and therapeutic implications. Science, 256, 774–779.
Coon, H., Byerley, W., Holik, J., et al. (1993). Linkage analysis of schizophrenia with five dopamine receptor genes in nine pedigrees. American Journal of Human Genetics, 52, 327–334.
Cooperative Human Linkage Center (CHLC)/Centre D'Etude Polymorphisme Humain (CEPH). (1994). A comprehensive human linkage map with centimorgan density. Science, 265, 2049.
Corder, E. H., Saunders, A. M., Strittmatter, W. J., et al. (1993). Gene dose of apolipoprotein E type 4 allele and the risk of Alzheimer's disease in the late onset families. Science, 261, 921–923.
Crocq, M. A., Mant, R., Asherson, P., et al. (1992). Association between schizophrenia and homozygosity at the dopamine D_3 receptor gene. Journal of Medical Genetics, 29, 858–860.

Davies, J. L., Kawaguchi, Y., Bennett, S. T., et al. (1994). A genome-wide search for human type I diabetes susceptibility genes. Nature, 371, 130–136.

de la Chapelle, A. (1993). Disease gene mapping in isolated human populations: The example of Finland. Journal of Medical Genetics, 30, 857–865.

Egeland, J. A., Gerhard, D. S., & Pauls, D. L. (1987). Bipolar affective disorders linked to DNA markers on chromosome 11. Nature, 325, 783–787.

Elston, R. C. (1994). P values, power, and pitfalls in the linkage analysis of psychiatric disorders. In E. S. Gershon & C. R. Cloninger (Eds.), Genetic approaches to mental disorders (pp. 3–21). Washington, DC: American Psychiatric Press.

Foucault, M. (1965). Madness and civilization: A history of insanity in the age of reason. New York: Random House.

Garrod, A. E. (1902). The incidence of alkaptonuria: A study of chemical individuality. Lancet, 2, 1616–1620.

Garver, K. L., & Garver, B. (1991). Feature article historical perspectives. Eugenics: Past, present, and the future. American Journal of Human Genetics, 49, 1109–1118.

Gelernter, J., Goldman, D., & Risch, N. (1993). The A1 allele at the D_2 dopamine receptor gene and alcoholism: A reappraisal. Journal of the American Medical Association, 269, 1673–1677.

George, V. T., Elston, R. C., Amos, C. I., et al. (1987). Association between polymorphic blood markers and risk factors for cardiovascular disease in a large pedigree. Genetic Epidemiology, 4, 267–275.

Goate, A., Chartier-Harlen, M. C., Mullan, M., et al. (1991). Segregation of a missense mutation in the amyloid precursor protein gene with familial Alzheimer's disease. Nature, 349, 704–706.

Goston, L. (1991). Genetic discrimination: The use of genetically based diagnosis and prognostic tests by employers and insurers. American Journal of Law and Medicine, 17, 109–144.

Hager, J., Hansen, L., Vaisse, C., et al. (1995). A missense mutation in the glucagon receptor gene is associated with non-insulin-dependent diabetes mellitus. Nature Genetics, 9, 299–304.

Hastbacka, J., de la Chapelle, A., Kaitila, I., et al. (1992). Linkage disequilibrium mapping in isolated founder populations: Diastrophic dysplasia in Finland. Nature Genetics, 2, 204–211.

Hoffman, E. P., Brown, R. H., Jr., & Kunkel, L. M. (1987). The protein product of the Duchenne muscular dystrophy locus. Cell, 51, 191–192.

Houwen, R. H. J., Baharloo, S., Blankenship, K., et al. (1994). Genome screening by searching for shared segments: Mapping a gene for benign recurrent intrahepatic cholestasis. Nature Genetics, 8, 380–386.

Hyde, T. M., Ziegler, J. C., & Weinberger, D. R. (1992). Psychiatric disturbances in metachromatic leukodystrophy: Insights into the neurobiology of psychosis. Archives of Neurology, 49, 401–406.

Jorde, L. B. (1995). Invited editorial: Linkage disequilibrium as a gene-mapping tool. American Journal of Genetics, 56, 11–14.

Kelsoe, J. R., Ginns, E. I., Egeland, J. A., et al. (1989). Re-evaluation of the linkage relationship between chromosome 11p loci and the gene for bipolar affective disorder in the Old Order Amish. Nature, 342, 238–243.

Kendler, K. S., & Eaves, L. J. (1986). Models for joint effect of genotype and environment on liability to psychiatric illness. American Journal of Psychiatry, 143, 279–289.

Kendler, K. S., Heath, A. C., Martin, N. G., et al. (1987). Symptoms of anxiety and symptoms of depression: Same genes, different environments? Archives of General Psychiatry, 44, 451–457.

Kennedy, J. L., Guiffra, L. A., Moises, H. W., *et al.* (1988). Evidence against linkage of schizophrenia to markers on chromosomes 5 in a northern Swedish pedigree. *Nature, 336,* 167–170.

Kuhn, T. S. (1970). *The structure of scientific revolutions* (2nd ed.). Chicago: University of Chicago Press.

Lander, E. S., & Schork, N. (1994). Genetic dissection of complex traits. *Science, 265,* 2037–2047.

Leiter, E. H., Coleman, D. L., & Hummel, K. P. (1981). The influence of genetic background on the expression of mutations at the diabetes locus in the mouse. III. Effect of H-2 haplotype and sex. *Diabetes, 30,* 1029–1034.

Lisitsyn, N., Lisitsyn, N., & Wigler, M. (1993). Cloning the difference between two complex genomes. *Science, 259,* 946–951.

Lisitsyn, N. A., Segre, J. A., Kusumi, K., *et al.* (1994). Direct isolation of polymorphic markers linked to a trait by genetically directed representational difference analysis. *Nature Genetics, 6,* 57–63.

Lyonnet, S., Bolino, A., Pelet, A., *et al.* (1993). A gene for Hirschsprung disease maps to the proximal long arm of chromosome 10. *Nature Genetics, 3,* 346.

McInnis, M. G., McMahon, F. J., Chase, G. A., *et al.* (1993). Anticipation in bipolar affective disorder. *American Journal of Human Genetics, 53,* 385–390.

McKusick, V. A. (1992). *Mendelian inheritance in man. Catalogs of autosomal dominant, autosomal recessive, and x-linked phenotypes.* (10th ed.). Baltimore: Johns Hopkins University Press.

MacLean, C. J., Ploughman, L. M., Diehl, S., *et al.* (1992). A new test for linkage in the presence of locus heterogeneity. *American Journal of Human Genetics, 50,* 1259–1266.

Miki, Y., Swensen, J., Shattuck-Eidens, D., *et al.* (1994). Isolation of BRCA1, the 17q linked breast and ovarian cancer susceptibility gene. *Science, 266,* 66–71.

Moldin, S. O., Gottesman, I. I., Erlenmeyer-Kimling, L., *et al.* (1990). Psychometric deviance in offspring at risk for schizophrenia, I: Initial delineation of a distinct subgroup. *Psychiatry Research, 32,* 297–310.

National Diabetes Data Group International Workgroup. (1979). Classification of diabetes mellitus and other categories of glucose intolerance. *Diabetes, 28,* 1039–1057.

Nelson, S. F., *et al.* (1993). Genomic mismatch scanning: A new approach to genetic linkage mapping. *Nature Genetics, 4,* 11.

Pacek, P., Sajantila, A., Syvanen, A. C. (1993). Determination of allele frequencies at loci with length polymorphism by quantitative analysis of DNA amplified from pooled samples. *PCR Methods and Applications, 2,* 313–317.

Paigen, K. (1995). A miracle enough: The power of mice. *Nature Medicine, 1,* 215–220.

Pakstis, A. J., Heutink, P., Pauls, D. L., *et al.* (1991). Progress in the search for genetic linkage with Tourette syndrome: An exclusion map covering more than 50% of the autosomal genome. *American Journal of Human Genetics, 48,* 281–294.

Pardes, H., Kaufmann, C. A., Pincus, H. A., *et al.* (1989). Genetics and psychiatry: Past discoveries, current dilemmas, and future directions. *American Journal of Psychiatry, 146,* 435–443.

Passarge, D. (1993). Wither polygenic inheritance: Mapping Hirschsprung disease. *Nature Genetics, 4,* 325.

Pauls, D. L. (1993). Behavioral disorders: Lessons in linkage. *Nature Genetics, 3,* 4–5.

Puffenberger, E. G., Kauffman, E. R., Bolk, S., *et al.* (1994). Identity-by-descent and association mapping of a recessive gene for Hirschsprung disease on human chromosome 13q22. *Human Molecular Genetics 3,* 1217–1225.

Pulver, A. E., Karayiorgou, M., Wolyniec, P. S., *et al.* (1994). Sequential strategy to identify

4

a susceptibility gene for schizophrenia: Report of potential linkage on chromosome 22q12–q13.1: Part 1. *American Journal of Medical Genetics, 54*, 36–43.

Reiss, D., Plomin, R., & Hetherington, E. M. (1991). Genetics and psychiatry: An unheralded window on the environment. *American Journal of Psychiatry, 148*, 283–291.

Rice, J. P., Reich, T., Andreasen, N. C., et al. (1987). The estimation of diagnostic sensitivity using stability data: An application to major depressive disorder. *Journal of Psychiatric Research, 21*, 337–345.

Risch, N. (1990). Linkage strategies for genetically complex traits, I: Multilocus models. *American Journal of Human Genetics, 46*, 222–228.

Romeo, G., Ronchetto, P., Luo, Y., et al. (1994). Point mutations affecting the tyrosine kinase domain of the RET proto-oncogene in Hirschsprung's disease. *Nature, 367*, 377–378.

Rotter, J. I., Vadheim, G. M., & Rimoin, D. L. (1992). Diabetes mellitus. In R. A. King, J. I. Rotter, & A. G. Motulsky (Eds.), *The genetic basis of common diseases* (pp. 413–481). London: Oxford University Press.

Schellenberg, G. D., Bird, T. D., Wijsman, E. M., et al. (1992). Genetic linkage evidence for a familial Alzheimer's disease locus on chromosome 14. *Science, 258*, 668–671.

Sherrington, R., Brynjolfsson, J., Petursson, H., et al. (1988). Localization of a susceptibility locus for schizophrenia on chromosome 5. *Nature, 336*, 164–167.

Solimena, M., & De Camilli, P. (1995). Coxsackieviruses and diabetes. *Nature Medicine, 1*, 25–26.

St George-Hyslop, P., Haines, J., Rogaev, E., et al. (1992). Genetic evidence for a novel familial Alzheimer's disease locus on chromosome 14. *Nature Genetics, 2*, 330–334.

Straub, R. E., Lehner, T., Luo, Y., et al. (1994). A possible vulnerability locus for bipolar affective disorder on chromosome 21q22.3. *Nature Genetics, 8*, 291–296.

Suarez, B. K., Hampe, C. L., & van Eerdewegh, P. (1994). Problems in replicating linkage claim in psychiatry. In E. S. Gershon & C. R. Cloninger (Eds.), *Genetic approaches to mental disorders* (pp. 23–46). Washington, DC: American Psychiatric Press.

Todd, J. A., Aitman, T. J., Cornall, R. J., et al. (1991). Genetic analysis of autoimmune type 1 diabetes mellitus in mice. *Nature 351*, 542.

Tsuang, M. T., & Lyons, M. J. (1989). Drawing the boundary of the schizophrenia spectrum: Evidence from a family study. In S. C. Schulz & C. A. Tamminga (Eds.), *Schizophrenia: Scientific progress* (pp. 23–27). New York: Oxford University Press.

Waldo, M. C., Carey, G., Myles-Worsley, M., et al. (1991). Codistribution of a sensory gating deficit and schizophrenia in multi-affected families. *Psychiatry Research, 39*, 257–268.

Wallace, M. R., Marchuk, D. A., Andersen, L. B., et al. (1990). Type 1 neurofibromatosis gene: Identification of a large transcript disrupted in three NF1 patients. *Science, 249*, 181–186.

Weeks, D. E., & Lange, K. (1993). The affected pedigree member method of linkage analysis. *American Journal of Human Genetics, 42*, 315–326.

Wooster, R., Neuhausen, S. L., Mangion, Y., et al. (1994). Localization of a breast cancer susceptibility gene, BRCA2, to chromosome 13q12–13. *Science, 265*, 2088–2090.

Zhang, Y., Proenca, R., Maffei, M., et al. (1994). Postional cloning of the mouse obese gene and its human homologue. *Nature, 372*, 425–432.

Zlotnik, L. H., Elston, R. C., & Namboodiri, K. K. (1983). Pedigree discriminant analysis: A method to identify monogenic segregation. *American Journal of Medical Genetics, 15*, 307–313.

CHAPTER 3

Beyond Nature versus Nurture

ROBERT PLOMIN

Shakespeare first brought the words *nature* and *nurture* together in *The Tempest,* when Prospero describes Caliban as "a devil on whose nature nurture can never stick." The idea of nature in conflict with nurture was the impetus for the alliterative phrase *nature–nurture,* used by Darwin's cousin, Francis Galton (1865), more than a century ago. Galton argued that "there is no escape from the conclusion that nature prevails enormously over nurture" (1883, p. 241). Joining these two words created a fission that exploded into the longest-lived controversy in the behavioral sciences. The dash in *nature–nurture* connoted the implicit conjunction "versus."

The purpose of this chapter is to show that the appropriate conjunction between *nature* and *nurture* is "and." The time has come to go beyond the *nature versus nurture* controversy. Genetic and environmental research strategies need to be brought together in order to understand the developmental duet between nature and nurture by which genotypes become phenotypes.

NATURE VERSUS NURTURE

During the past century, the pendulum has swung back and forth several times between nature and nurture. A pessimist's view of these swings is that they are becoming faster, wider, and more divisive. Figure 1 presents my optimistic view that the pendulum is losing its inertia and is

ROBERT PLOMIN • Institute of Psychiatry, London SE5 8AF, United Kingdom.
Genetics and Mental Illness: Evolving Issues for Research and Society, edited by Laura Lee Hall. Plenum Press, New York, 1996.

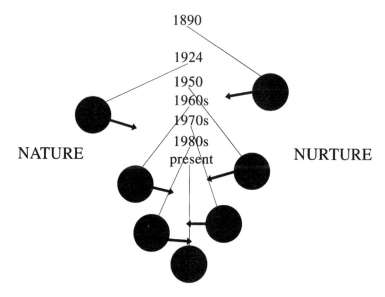

Figure 1.   Swings of the nature–nurture pendulum in American psychology.

coming to rest in between nature and nurture. The figure is meant to be seen as a pendulum swinging back and forth as you proceed down in time. This is my subjective view of nature and nurture in American psychology during the past century. It begins in 1890 with the publication of William James's *Principles of Psychology,* a book that provided the agenda for much psychological research but scarcely mentioned individual differences or heredity. It is critically important to recognize that behavioral genetic research is limited to the investigation of the genetic and environmental origins of individual differences within a species, not species-typical development. Its focus is on genetic and environmental factors that make a difference in behavioral dimensions and disorders. That is, its genetic focus is on DNA differences among individuals, not the vast majority of DNA that is the same for all members of a species. The word does not connote the *nature* of the human species, for example. Specifically, *nature* refers to *inheritance,* DNA differences transmitted from generation to generation. Many DNA events are not inherited and thus are not counted as "genetic" in this sense. For example, Down syndrome is caused by a chromosomal abnormality but in most cases it is not inherited and thus not counted as genetic. Similarly, the word *nurture* also refers just to differences among individuals, not to the many environmental factors such as nutrients, light, and oxygen that do not vary or are functionally equivalent among members of a species. However, in contrast to the very restricted use of the word *nature* in behavioral genetics, the word *nurture* is used very broadly. Basically, *nurture* is used to refer to any effects on individual differences in behavior than are not inherited. Thus, nurture includes any nongenetic processes such as perinatal events, illness, and diet as well as psychosocial processes. As is the case for any definition, these definitions of *nature* and *nurture* are arbitrary. In order to interpret behavioral genetic research, however, it is important to recognize that such research only addresses sources of differences among individuals in a population and that the word *nature* is used in a restricted sense.

Galton's enthusiasm for the importance of nature over nurture, riding the crest of the wave created by his cousin Darwin and the rediscovery of Mendel's laws of inheritance, kindled interest in heredity during the first few decades of this century. The first twin and adoption studies of behavior were reported in 1924, for example. This represented a swing from a naive environmentalism in which the notion that all men are created equal was misinterpreted to mean that all men are created identical, a misinterpretation that continues to be a core misunderstanding about genetic influence today. The signers of the U.S. Declaration of Independence clearly did not mean that there are no important differences among people. What they meant is that all people should be equal in rights and before the law. The fundamental need for a democracy is to treat people equally *despite* their differences. Even John Locke, whose writings on the *tabula rasa* and the importance of experience inspired the American and French revolutions, understood that people are inherently different (Loehlin, 1983).

This swing toward nature also includes eugenics, a word coined by Galton. Both came to an abrupt halt with the misguided eugenic policies of the Nazis. Such political forces curbing the shift toward nature have often been discussed (e.g., Kevles, 1985). In psychology, this swing back to nurture also coincided with the emergence of behaviorism. Behaviorism arose in the 1920s as a protest against all forms of "introspective psychology," which was concerned with mental states such as consciousness and will. The term *behaviorism* refers to a strict focus on observable behavioral responses. Because its emphasis on observable responses also led to an emphasis on observable environmental stimuli, behaviorism came to imply *environmentalism*. Stimulus–response chains eventually became the only acceptable explanation of behavior. Behaviorism also moved in the direction of environmentalism with its rejection of the instinct doctrine of McDougall (1908). At that time, instincts were thought of as inherited patterns of behavior, and the behaviorists attacked this position as circular. However, in rejecting this naive view of instincts, the behaviorists also discarded the notion that heredity can influence behavior.

These trends led J. B. Watson, the founder of behaviorism, to issue his frequently quoted challenge:

> Give me a dozen healthy infants and my own specified world to bring them up in, and I'll guarantee to take any one at random and train him to become any type of specialist I might select—doctor, lawyer, artist, merchant-chief and, yes, even beggar and thief, regardless of his talents, penchants, tendencies, abilities, vocations, and race of his ancestors. [Watson, 1924, p. 104]

During the 1940s and 1950s, behaviorism and learning theory dominated American psychology. For mental illness, this was fertile ground for Freud's brand of environmentalism that blamed psychopathology on parental treatment during the first few years of life (Torrey, 1992). Nonetheless, by 1960, there were signs that the pendulum was swinging back toward nature. Research on animal behavior such as studies comparing inbred strains of mice and artificial selection experiments provided powerful demonstrations of the importance of genetics on behavior. The trickle of human behavioral genetic research that had begun in the 1920s with twin and adoption studies continued but remained outside the mainstream of the behavioral sciences. This work, especially the animal research, led to the first behavioral genetics textbook in 1960 (Fuller & Thompson, 1960).

In 1963 an influential article reviewed family, twin, and adoption data for IQ scores and concluded that genetic influence is important for this trait (Erlenmeyer-Kimling & Jarvik, 1963). In 1966 the classic adoption study of schizophrenia by Heston documented the influence of heredity in mental illness, a conclusion in line with previous twin studies. The genetics of mental illness was firmly established with the publication of *Genetic Theory and Abnormal Behavior* (Rosenthal, 1970) and *The Genetics of Mental Disorders* (Slater & Cowie, 1971). Thus, in the 1960s, some momentum had begun to build for genetic research in psychology and psychiatry. However, this momentum ended, especially in psychology, in 1969 when Arthur Jensen published a paper that reviewed the evidence for genetic influence on IQ scores and suggested that the average IQ difference between blacks and whites may in part be related to genetic differences. Jensen's article, combined with a book by Herrnstein (1973) suggesting genetic differences between classes, provoked a furious response unparalleled in the behavioral sciences until the current turmoil raised by Herrnstein and Murray's (1994) book that resurrects these issues. The reaction to Jensen and Herrnstein threatened the existence of the fledgling field of human behavioral genetics, even though very few behavioral geneticists studied racial or class differences. The furor subsided only gradually during the 1970s as the spotlight moved to new research on genetic influence on individual differences in mental illness, personality, and cognitive abilities.

In the 1980s, the pendulum again began to swing back toward nature, at least in part as a result of this new research and of the excitement caused by advances in molecular genetics. Even for IQ scores, one of the most controversial areas in behavioral genetics, a 1987 survey of more than a 1000 social and behavioral scientists and educators indicated that most had accepted a significant role for heredity (Snyderman & Rothman, 1987). For mental illness, the message for the 1960s was that nature is important. By the 1980s, the message was that mental illness is not entirely related to nature.

The reason for hoping that the pendulum is coming to rest at a point in between nature and nurture is not that we want everyone to be happy. It is what genetic research tells us.

BEYOND DEMONSTRATIONS OF THE IMPORTANCE OF NATURE

In the 1950s and 1960s, most behavioral genetic research merely set out to show that heredity contributes to behavior in order to counteract the widespread environmentalism of the times. Evidence for at least some genetic influence has been found for most behavioral dimensions and disorders that have been investigated (McGuffin, Owen, O'Donovan, Thapar, & Gottesman, 1994; Plomin, DeFries, & McClearn, 1990). For example, identical and fraternal twin probandwise concordances are, respectively, about 45 and 15% for schizophrenia, about 65 and 25% for major affective disorders, and about 60 and 10% for autism (Plomin, Owen, & McGuffin, 1994). Adoption data generally confirm the twin results. More research of this type is still needed to answer the rudimentary question of whether and how much genetic factors contribute to components and constellations of behavioral disorders. For example, the assumption that alcoholism is highly heritable was so strong that only recently have large-scale twin studies been conducted. These studies find only moderate heritability for males and very modest heritability for females (McGue, 1993). Identical and fraternal twin concordances are, respectively, about 40 and 20% in males and about 30 and 25% in females. Basic genetic research is needed to investigate whether genetic influence is stronger for certain components of alcohol abuse, such as sensitivity to alcohol, or for certain constellations, e.g., alcohol abuse coupled with personality disorders such as undercontrol or with cognitive factors such as certain attitudes about alcohol use.

However, we have reached the point at which it is shortsighted to conduct genetic research merely to demonstrate genetic influence on yet another dimension or disorder. It is a safe assumption that some genetic influence will be found. What is needed now is research that goes beyond the questions of whether and how much genetic factors contribute to a disorder. Three examples that can be addressed in quantitative genetic research such as twin and adoption studies include developmental genetic analysis, multivariate genetic analysis, and analysis of the genetic links between the normal and abnormal. An obvious direction, of course, is to use the new tools of molecular genetics to begin to identify genes responsible for heritability. Later in this chapter, another important direction for research will be discussed, namely combining genetic and environmental research strategies in order to study the interplay between nature and nurture in the development of mental illness.

Developmental Genetic Analysis

The strength and nature of genetic effects can change during development (Plomin, 1986). Concerning the strength of genetic effects, heritability can change as the relative magnitude of genetic or environmental factors changes during development. Although it is reasonable to assume that environmental factors become increasingly important as experiences accumulate during life, research on cognitive ability shows that genetic factors increase almost linearly in importance during the life span (McGue, Bouchard, Iacono, & Lykken, 1993). This could occur, for example, if individuals increasingly seek out environments that foster their genetic propensities, i.e., active genotype–environment correlation. For mental illness, such developmental comparisons are rare. For example, little is known about the genetic and environmental origins of depression before adulthood (Lombroso, Pauls, & Leckman, 1994; Rutter et al., 1990). A second type of developmental genetic analysis investigates genetic contributions to change across time using longitudinal data. That is, to what extent do genetic effects at one age differ from genetic effects at another age? For example, to what extent do genetic effects on depression differ from adolescence to young adulthood to middle adulthood to late adulthood?

Multivariate Genetic Analysis

Multivariate genetic analysis assesses genetic contributions to covariance among dimensions and disorders rather than to the variance of each considered separately. That is, to what extent do genetic effects on one disorder also affect another disorder? Multivariate genetic analysis can address the fundamental issues of heterogeneity and comorbidity for psychiatric disorders, contributing to a nosology at the level of etiology rather than at the level of symptoms.

The essence of assessing genetic and environmental contributions to phenotypic covariance is the cross-correlation or cross-concordance. For example, a cross-twin correlation is the correlation between one twin's score on one measure and the other twin's score on the other measure. Everything else is similar to the usual univariate analysis of the variance of a single measure. If, for example, cross-twin correlations between two measures are greater for identical twins than for fraternal twins, this suggests that genetic factors contribute to the correlation between the traits. Taking into account the heritability of the two traits, it is possible to estimate the extent of genetic overlap between the two traits. For example, for cognitive ability and scholastic achievement, several recent studies found that genetic effects overlap completely (Wadsworth, 1994). For behavior problems, similar results indicating genetic overlap have been reported for major depression and generalized anxiety disorder (Kendler, Neale, Kessler, Heath, & Eaves, 1992), major depression and phobias (Kendler, Neale, Kessler, Heath, & Eaves, 1993), and major depression and alcoholism (Kendler, Heath, Neale, Kessler, & Eaves, 1993). Comorbid conditions may be the rule rather than the exception for many domains of psychopathology (Caron & Rutter, 1991), and genetics appears to be the source of such comorbidity (Plomin & Rende, 1991).

Links between the Normal and Abnormal

If multiple genes are responsible for genetic influences on behavioral dimensions and disorders, a continuum of genetic risk is likely to extend from normal to abnormal behavior. New methods have been developed to address this fundamental issue (DeFries & Fulker, 1985, 1988; Eaves et al., 1993). For example, reading disability appears to represent the genetic extreme of a continuous distribution (DeFries & Gillis, 1993). In other words, genetic effects on reading disability appear to be merely the genetic extreme of a continuum of genetic effects on reading ability. It has been proposed that much mental illness will also show strong genetic links between the normal and abnormal (Plomin, 1991). Two twin studies of attention-deficit hyperactivity disorder (ADHD) indicate that strong genetic factors affect both the dimension of ADHD-related symptoms and extreme scores (Gillis, Gilger, Pennington, & DeFries, 1992; Stevenson, 1992). However, one such analysis of adolescent depressive symptoms found moderate genetic influence for the full range of individual differences in depression

but negligible genetic influence on extreme scores (Rende, Plomin, Reiss, &
Hetherington, 1993).

Identifying Specific Genes Responsible for Heritability

Molecular genetics holds great promise for moving beyond the mere
demonstration of genetic influence to identifying specific genes. Although
these techniques can find the chromosomal location of any single-gene
effect, the task of finding specific genes in complex systems influenced by
multiple genes as well as multiple environmental factors is much more
difficult (Plomin, Owen, & McGuffin, 1994). The best behavioral example
so far is the repeatedly replicated association between late-onset Alzheimer's disease and a particular allele (the E4 allele) of the apolipoprotein
gene (Apo), one of the genes responsible for cholesterol transport. The
presence of this Apo-E4 allele increases risk about sixfold for late-onset
Alzheimer's disease.

For other behavioral disorders, most notably for schizophrenia and
bipolar affective disorder, early reports of linkage to chromosomal regions
did not replicate. However, these studies were based on research designs
that could only detect a major gene effect necessary and sufficient to develop
the disorder. Indeed, it may be unlikely that major-gene effects are responsible for the heritability of such complex disorders. Newer techniques can
detect genes of relatively small effect size that contribute probabilistically
and interchangeably to mental illness.

NURTURE AS WELL AS NATURE

In order to make sure that the pendulum illustrated in Figure 1 does
not swing too far toward nature given the allure of molecular genetics,
it should be emphasized that genetic research not only indicates genetic
influence but also provides the best available evidence for the importance
of environmental influence. For example, the concordance of identical twins
for schizophrenia is about 45%. This means that as often as not, these
pairs of genetically identical individuals are discordant for schizophrenia
as currently diagnosed. There can be no genetic explanation for this dis-
cordance and it provides evidence for the powerful role of environmental
factors. It should be noted that the "environment" in genetic research
denotes all nonheritable factors, including possible biological experiences
such as prenatal events and postnatal illness and even nontransmissible
stochastic DNA events, in addition to possible psychosocial experiences.

It really means *nongenetic,* which is a much broader definition of the word *environment* than is usually encountered.

For unipolar depression, the concordance for identical twins is also about 45%, again suggesting substantial environmental influence. For conduct disorder, identical twin concordance is much higher, about 85%, but fraternal twin concordance is also high, about 70%, again suggesting substantial environmental influence. Two exceptions to the rule that nongenetic factors are at least as important as genetic factors in mental illness may be manic-depressive disorder and autism. Although not studied nearly as extensively as schizophrenia, manic-depressive disorder appears to yield identical and fraternal twin concordances of about 65 and 20%, respectively. For autism, concordances are about 65% for identical twins and 10% for fraternal twins (Rutter, Bailey, Bolton, & Le Couteur, 1993). Even these two counterexamples, however, imply the presence of some nongenetic influence for these two disorders because about 35% of pairs of identical twins are discordant.

A technical aside is necessary at this point to explain why heritabilities for mental illness are often reported to be very much higher than implied by these concordances for identical twins. Concordances are based on dichotomous data such as a diagnosis of an individual as affected or not. Such dichotomous concordance data are not amenable to estimating heritability, which refers to continuous variation in a population. For this reason, concordances are converted to a type of correlation (tetrachoric correlation) that assumes an underlying continuum of liability even though the concordance data are dichotomous (Falconer, 1965). That is, although the basic data consist of a dichotomous diagnosis of affected or not affected, they are converted based on the assumption that there is a continuum of risk from the normal to the abnormal. These concordances-converted-to-correlations are then used to calculate a statistic called the heritability of liability. Estimates of the heritability of liability usually suggest greater genetic influence than do the concordances themselves. For example, for schizophrenia, estimates of the heritability of liability sometimes exceed 80%, even though the concordance for identical twins is less than 50%. It is important to emphasize that the heritability of liability refers to a hypothetical construct of an underlying continuous liability toward a disorder, not to the disorder as diagnosed (Plomin, 1991). There is good reason to believe that multiple-gene influences on complex disorders result in continuous dimensions rather than dichotomous disorders. However, it is important to assess such continuous dimensions directly rather than to assume them from dichotomous diagnoses.

The reason for discussing this technical issue is its relevance to the argument that the pendulum in Figure 1 really is coming to rest at a point between nature and nurture. Unless environmental researchers respect the growing evidence for the importance of genetic factors, the results of their research will continue to be causally ambiguous. For example, studying environmental factors in families whose members are genetically related leaves open the possibility that associations between family environment and children's adjustment are mediated genetically rather than environmentally. On the other hand, unless genetic researchers respect the importance of environmental factors, their research will not go beyond the rudimentary nature–nurture questions of whether and how much genetic influence is important. The molecular genetic search for genes will also profit by using environmentally sophisticated designs. At the least, measures of the environment need to be incorporated into behavioral genetic studies. The key questions concern the developmental interplay between nature and nurture.

Investigating nurture may be even more difficult than investigating nature. For environmental transmission, there is nothing comparable to the laws of hereditary transmission or to the gene as a basic unit of transmission. How is the environment transmitted and translated? What are the units of environmental transmission? Although much remains to be learned about genetics, understanding of genetic processes seems to be light-years ahead of our understanding of environmental processes. As a sign of the utility of integrating genetic and environmental research strategies, two of the most novel and far-reaching discoveries about the environment in recent years come from genetic research: the importance of nonshared environment and the role of genetics in experience.

NONSHARED ENVIRONMENT

Behavioral genetic research consistently suggests that the salient environmental influences in development operate to make children growing up in the same family no more similar than children growing up in different families. That is, salient environmental influences are not shared by children growing up in the same family. This revolutionary finding of the importance of nonshared environment lay hidden in behavioral genetic research for decades because behavioral geneticists focused on the genetic results of their research. However, human quantitative genetic methods have always separated environmental variance into two components. One component, called *shared* or *common environmental variance,* involves environmental influences that contribute to familial resemblance. The goal of quantitative genetic designs is to disentangle this environmental contribution to familial resemblance from the genetic contribution to familial resemblance. The other component of environmental variance refers to the rest of the environmental variance, environmental variance that does not contribute to familial resemblance. It is called nonshared environmental variance in the sense that it is defined as environmental variance that is not of the shared variety.

Shared environmental variance can be estimated directly from the correlation between genetically unrelated children adopted together, called *adoptive siblings*. The resemblance of adoptive siblings can only be the result of shared family environment, not of shared heredity. Shared environment can also be estimated, albeit much less directly and powerfully, from twin designs. The twin design estimates shared environment as the extent to which identical twin resemblance cannot be explained by genetic resemblance. Specifically, shared environment is estimated as the difference between the identical twin correlation and heritability.

Because both adoption and twin designs estimate variance related to heritability and to shared environment, nonshared environment can be estimated as variance not explained by heritability or by shared environment. In the twin design, nonshared environment can also be estimated in terms of differences within pairs of identical twins. Identical twins are identical genetically and thus differences within pairs cannot be related to genetic factors, as mentioned earlier. More specifically, differences within pairs of identical twins are related to nonshared environment plus error of measurement. Error of measurement needs to be considered in the context of nonshared environment because family members, including identical twins, differ for reasons of error of measurement as well as for reasons of reliable nonshared environmental influences.

The overview of twin results mentioned earlier to demonstrate the importance of environmental influences also indicates the importance of nonshared environment. The most direct evidence for the importance of nonshared environment comes from the low concordances for identical twins. For example, for schizophrenia, unipolar depression, and alcoholism, identical twin concordances less than 50% suggest not only that environmental factors are important but also that environmental factors are of the nonshared variety. As mentioned, manic-depression and autism appear to show greater genetic influence than these other disorders. However, environmental influences involved in manic-depression and autism also appear to be exclusively of the nonshared type. For all of these domains, studies of adoptive siblings are needed to provide more direct tests of the importance of shared environment. Although twin data for conduct disorder appear to suggest the presence of shared environmental influence because concordances for both identical and fraternal twins are high, this may not be the case. It has been suggested that both types of twins are so similar for conduct disorder because they are partners in crime (Rowe, 1983a).

Nonshared environment also accounts for nearly all environmental influence for self-reported personality and for cognitive abilities after childhood. Evidence for the importance of nonshared environment for behavioral development has been summarized elsewhere (Plomin, Chipuer, & Neiderhiser, 1994; Plomin & Daniels, 1987). Nonshared environment is also critical for common medical disorders and physical traits (Dunn & Plomin, 1990).

Despite the novelty and far-reaching implications of the conclusion that environmental influences relevant to mental illness are largely of the nonshared variety, I am aware of no major criticisms of these findings or their interpretation. It is rare in a field as complex as the behavioral sciences to discover such clear and consistent evidence for a finding that radically alters the way we think about an issue as basic as the influence of the family on development. So often it has been assumed that the key environmental influences on children's development are shared by siblings: their parents' personality and childhood experiences, the quality of their parents' marital relationships, their parents' educational background and socioeconomic status, the neighborhood in which they grow up, and their parents' attitude to school or to discipline. Yet to the extent that these influences are shared by children growing up in the same family, they cannot account for the differences we observe in mental illness.

Not only does the discovery of the importance of nonshared environment suggest what is wrong with our previous environmental approaches to children's development, it also points to what needs to be done. We need to identify environmental factors that make two children growing up in the same family so different from one another. The message is not that family experiences are unimportant but rather that the relevant environmental influences are specific to each child, not general to an entire family. These findings suggest that instead of thinking about children's environments on a family-by-family basis, we need to think about environments on an individual-by-individual basis. The critical question is, why are children in the same family so different? Answers to this question are the key that can unlock the secrets of environmental influence on the development of all children, not just siblings.

To address the question of why children in the same family are so different, it is obviously necessary to study more than one child per family. Three steps in research on nonshared environment are needed: (1) identify environmental influences specific to each child that are not shared by siblings; (2) identify sibling differences in experience that predict differences in outcomes; and (3) disentangle cause and effect (Plomin, 1994a). Considerable progress has been made on the first step. Many measures of the environment that have been employed in developmental research are general to a family rather than specific to a child. For example, if we simply ask whether or not parents have been divorced, this is the same for two children in the family. Assessed in this family-general manner, divorce cannot be a source of differences in siblings' outcomes because it does not differ for two children in the same family. However, research on divorce has shown that divorce affects children in a family differently (Hetherington & Clingempeel, 1992). If divorce is assessed in a child-specific manner that can capture differential experiences of siblings, it could well be a source of differential sibling outcomes.

Thus, the first advantage of thinking about environmental influences from the perspective of nonshared environment is that it forces us to develop child-specific measures of the environment. Even when environmental measures are specific to a child, they can be shared by two children in a family. For example, observations of a mother's affection toward a child are specific to that child, but to what extent are affectionate mothers affectionate in equal measure to two children? It is not possible to predict *a priori* which aspects of the environment are shared and which are not shared. Studies of siblings are needed to identify nonshared environmental factors. Research so far suggests that children growing up in the same family experience surprisingly different environments if you ask them about their experiences or if you observe them interacting with family members, but not if you ask their parents. Children growing up in the same family in fact experience quite different family environments, so much so that a book on this topic is called *Separate Lives: Why Siblings are so Different* (Dunn & Plomin, 1990). Children are exquisitely sensitive to differential parental treatment, even from a very early age (Dunn & Munn, 1985). Outside the family, siblings can also lead very different lives, especially in relation to their peers and friends.

In summary, research on nonshared environment has begun to identify environmental influences that are specific to each child in a family and not shared by siblings. The next step is to investigate the extent to which nonshared environmental candidates predict particular outcomes of children. That is, there can be no guarantee that a specific nonshared environmental measure will be responsible for nonshared environmental variance for a particular outcome measure. Although it is very early in this research, some success has been achieved in predicting differences in adjustment outcomes from sibling differences in experiences (Hetherington, Reiss, & Plomin, 1994). One early plot line that is emerging is a dark story in which differential negative behavior of parents relates to adolescents' negative outcomes such as antisocial behavior and depression, whereas differences in positive behavior of parents seem less important (Reiss *et al.,* in press). Although it makes sense to investigate systematic sources of nonshared environment such as differential parenting, we need to keep our minds open to the possibility that chance can also contribute to nonshared environment in the sense of idiosyncratic experiences or the subtle interplay of a concatenation of events (Dunn & Plomin, 1990).

The best hope for such research is that it will uncover new nonshared environmental processes that predict important developmental outcomes and that have not been considered in traditional between-family environmental research. If reality falls short of this ideal, nonshared environmental research will at least be valuable as a crucible for family research. That is, unless a family variable can be shown to operate within families, in the sense that it is experienced differently and has differential effects on children in the same family, it cannot be an important environmental predictor of developmental outcomes.

Finally, when associations are found between nonshared environment and outcomes, the question of direction of effects is raised. Is differential parental treatment the cause or the effect of sibling differences in behavior? One way to begin to disentangle cause and effect is by means of longitudinal analyses. Another approach involves genetic research strategies. Nonshared experiences of siblings may reflect genetically-instigated differences between the siblings such as differences in temperament. This issue of genetic contributions to experience is a new development at the interface between genetics and environment.

THE ROLE OF GENETICS IN EXPERIENCE

This second genetic discovery about the environment has been called the nature of nurture (Plomin & Bergeman, 1991). During the past decade, many widely used measures of the environment have shown genetic influence in dozens of twin and adoption studies. Research with diverse twin and adoption experimental designs has found genetic influence on parenting, childhood accidents, television viewing, classroom environments, peer groups, social support, work environments, life events, divorce, exposure to drugs, education, and socioeconomic status (Plomin, 1994b).

How is it possible for a measure of the environment to show genetic influence? If one thinks about the environment as independent of the person, environmental measures obviously cannot show genetic influence. The weather might affect mood, but weather *per se* is not inherited. However, measures of the psychological environment are not independent of the person. Measures of psychological environments usually involve behavior of the individual. For example, measures of the family environment are not independent of the child. Parent–child interactions involve behavior of both children and parents and could by these routes show genetic influence. Experiences outside the family such as social support and life events can also be influenced by characteristics of the individual.

How can genetic influence on environmental measures be detected? The simple trick is to treat environmental measures as dependent measures in twin and adoption studies. If an environmental measure is not influenced by genetic factors, the correlation for identical twins will be no greater than correlations for fraternal twins, and correlations for genetically related family members will be no greater than correlations for genetically unrelated members of adoptive families. The surprising finding has been that twin and adoption studies consistently point to genetic influence on measures of the environment. Such findings suggest that environmental measures reflect genetic differences among individuals. This may best be construed as genotype–environment correlation in which genetic propensities are correlated with experiences.

The most recent data of this type come from the Nonshared Environment and Adolescent Development (NEAD) project, designed to identify specific sources of nonshared environment relevant to adolescent adjustment in the context of a genetically sensitive design (Reiss et al., in press). The NEAD samples includes 720 families with same-sex adolescent sibling pairs from 10 to 18 years of age from two types of families, never-divorced families and stepfamilies, with six types of siblings: identical twins, fraternal twins, and full siblings in never-divorced families, and full siblings, half siblings, and unrelated siblings in stepfamilies. The adolescents rated their mothers and fathers and parents rated themselves on 12 scales that assessed diverse aspects of family dynamics such as expression of affection, closeness, conflict, discipline, and monitoring.

Of the 12 scales, significant genetic effects were found for all but one scale (control) for adolescents' ratings of mother and for all but one scale (symbolic aggression during conflict) for ratings of father (Plomin, Reiss, Hetherington, & Howe, 1994). The average heritability estimates for the 12 scales were 30% for ratings of mother and 31% for ratings of father, suggesting that nearly a third of the total variance of these measures of family environment can be accounted for by genetic differences among children. Composite measures were derived from factor analyses of the 12 measures. Three factors emerged for adolescents' ratings of both mother and father: positive, negative, and control. Model-fitting heritability estimates for the three factors were 30, 40, and 29%, respectively, for ratings of mother, and 56, 23, and 46% for ratings of father. Similar results were found for parents' ratings of their own behavior toward each child, which is important because it suggests that genetic effects are not only in the heads of the adolescents.

In addition to these questionnaire measures, NEAD employed videotape observations of dyads (each parent with each child) engaged in 10-minute discussions around problems and conflicts relevant to the particular dyad. The behavior of each parent and each child in the four dyadic sessions was rated independently on 14 dimensions including warmth, self-disclosure, involvement, assertiveness, and control. These dimensions were incor-

porated in a measurement model as multiple indices of the same three
factors the parents' contributions to the interaction: positive, negative, and
control. Model-fitting analyses for error-corrected latent variables repre-
senting these factors yielded evidence for significant genetic influence for
all three factors for fathers' behavior toward their children and for all but
the control factor for mothers' behavior (O'Connor, Hetherington, Reiss, &
Plomin, in press). Heritability estimates for the positive, negative, and
control factors were 18, 24, and 24%, respectively, for fathers, and 18, 38,
and 0% for mothers.

Children's contributions to family interactions yielded greater heritability estimates than parents' contributions. For the children's contribution
to positive and negative interactions, heritability estimates were 64 and
52%, respectively, for interactions with fathers, and 59 and 48% for interactions with mothers. Greater heritability for children's as compared to parents' contributions to family interactions is related to the child-based genetic
design of NEAD in that the twins and siblings are children not parents. A
child-based genetic design can only detect genetic factors in parents' behavior that reflect genetically based behavioral differences among children. If
a similar study were conducted using a parent-based genetic design, such
as adult twins interacting with their children, greater heritabilities would
be expected for parental contributions to family interactions and lower
heritabilities for children's contributions.

These NEAD data confirm the results of more than a dozen earlier
studies using diverse designs that suggested genetic influences on a variety
of measures of family and extrafamilial environments (Plomin, 1994b). A
far-reaching implication is this: If measures of environment show genetic
influence and if measures of mental illness also show genetic influence,
then it is possible that genetic factors contribute in part to correlations
between environmental measures and measures of mental illness (Plomin,
1995). Stated more simply, genes can contribute to ostensibly nongenetic
influences on mental illness.

Although everyone knows that correlation does not imply causation,
correlations between environmental measures and mental illness are usually
interpreted as if the environmental measure caused the mental illness environmentally. The possibility of the alternative direction of effects, from
individual to environment, is considered in theory, especially in theories
of socialization and parent–child interactions (Russell & Russell, 1992),
although not nearly so often in practice. There is also a third alternative
explanation of a correlation between two factors, X and Y. Not only can
X cause Y, or Y cause X, but a third factor can be responsible for the
correlation between X and Y. Research showing the contribution of genetics
to experience suggests that genetics needs to be given serious consideration

as a possible "third factor" accounting in part for associations between environmental measures and mental illness.

This topic can be viewed as an attempt to identify genotype–environment correlation for specific measures of environment. Genotype–environment correlation literally refers to the correlation between genetic and environmental influences for a particular trait. Three types of genotype–environment correlation have been described: passive, reactive, and active (Plomin, DeFries, & Loehlin, 1977). Passive genotype–environment correlation occurs because parents share both genes and environment with their offspring. For this reason, children can passively inherit environments that are correlated with their genetic propensities. Reactive genotype–environment correlation refers to experiences of individuals that derive from reactions of other people to the individuals' genetic propensities. Active genotype–environment correlation occurs when individuals select, modify, construct, or reconstruct experiences that are correlated with their genetic propensities.

Three methods are available to investigate the contribution of genetic factors to correlations between environmental measures and mental illness. These methods differ in the type of genotype–environment correlation that they detect. The first method, comparing correlations between environmental measures and outcomes in nonadoptive and adoptive families, focuses on passive genotype–environment correlation. The second method considers reactive and active genotype–environment correlation by comparing experiences of adopted individuals with characteristics of their biological parents. The third method, a multivariate genetic analysis of correlations between environmental measures and outcomes, addresses all three types of genotype–environment correlation. These methods are described elsewhere (Plomin, 1994b). Such analyses show that genetic factors mediate environment–outcome associations to a surprising extent. For example, in NEAD, parental negativity correlates with adolescents' antisocial behavior and depressive symptoms largely for genetic reasons (Pike, McGuire, Hetherington, Reiss, & Plomin, in press). Such results provide the basis for the conclusion drawn earlier that genes can contribute to ostensibly nongenetic influences on mental illness. Other research suggests that genetics contributes to life events and social support as they relate to depression (Plomin, 1994b).

What are the implications of finding that genetic factors contribute to measures of environment and to correlations between environmental measures and adjustment? Two easily drawn implications are wrong. This research does *not* mean that environment is unimportant. Genetic research clearly indicates that most of the variance in environmental measures is not genetic in origin. However, the news is that widely used environmental measures show significant genetic influence. Second, these findings do *not* imply that clinicians are limited in their ability to intervene successfully. Heritability does not imply untreatability. For dimensions and disorders influenced by complex systems of mutliple genes and multiple environmental factors, genetic influence refers to probabilistic propensities rather than predetermined programming. However, a fundamental implication is that environmental measures cannot be assumed to be environmental just because they are called environmental. Indeed, research to date suggests that it is safer to assume that ostensible measures of the environment include genetic effects. Associations between measures of the environment and mental illness cannot be safely assumed to be purely environmental in origin. Taking this argument to the extreme, a recent book has concluded that socialization research in families of genetically related individuals is fundamentally flawed (Rowe, 1994).

Consideration of genetic contributions to measures of environment suggests new ways of thinking about environmental influences in development. For example, it provides an empirical basis for exploring children's active role in creating and interpreting their experience (Scarr, 1992). Environmental theory has moved away from passive models of development in favor of models that recognize the active role of individuals in selecting, modifying, and creating their own environments. Despite this shift in environmental theory, research seldom addresses the active role of individuals in creating their own environments. It seems likely that measures that assess individuals' active engagement with their environments will show even greater evidence for genetic influence. For example, research to date suggests that characteristics of adolescents' peer groups show greater heritability than measures of family environment. If this finding is replicated, it could occur because children select their peers and are selected by them.

NATURE AND NURTURE

The convergence of evidence from family, twin, and adoption studies makes it clear that genetics plays a major role in the origins of individual differences in mental illness. There is still much to be learned about the rudimentary nature–nurture questions of whether and how much genetic factors contribute to behavioral variation. However, the future of genetic research in psychology lies in going beyond these basic questions about heritability to take advantage of new developmental and multivariate techniques and methods to investigate genetic and environmental links between the normal and abnormal. The emerging ability to identify specific genes involved in complex behavior is a particularly exciting possibility that will revolutionize genetic research by making it possible to identify relevant genotypes directly for individuals.

Perhaps most important of all is the usefulness of genetic research strategies to investigate the environment, as seen in the examples of non-shared environment and genetic contributions to experience. Genetic research can tell us as much about nurture as about nature. It seems clear that some of the most interesting questions for genetic research involve the environment and some of the most interesting questions for environmental research involve genetics. Both genetic and environmental research on mental illness will profit from ensuring that the conjunction in the phrase *nature–nurture* is *and*—not *versus*.

REFERENCES

Caron, C., & Rutter, M. (1991). Comorbidity in child psychopathology: Concepts, issues, and research strategies. *Journal of Child Psychology and Psychiatry, 32,* 1063–1080.

DeFries, J. C., & Fulker, D. W. (1985). Multiple regression analysis of twin data. *Behavior Genetics, 15,* 467–473.

DeFries, J. C., & Fulker, D. W. (1988). Multiple regression analysis of twin data: Etiology of deviant scores versus individual differences. *Acta Geneticae Medicae et Gemellologiae, 37,* 205–216.

DeFries, J. C., & Gillis, J. C. (1993). Genetics of reading disability. In R. Plomin & G. E. McClearn (Eds.), *Nature, nurture, and psychology* (pp. 121–145). Washington, DC: American Psychological Association.

Dunn, J., & Munn, P. (1985). Becoming a family member: Family conflict and the development of social understanding. *Child Development, 56,* 480–492.

Dunn, J., & Plomin, R. (1990). *Separate lives: Why siblings are so different.* New York: Basic Books.

Eaves, L., Silberg, J., Hewitt, J. K., Meyer, J., Rutter, M., Simonoff, E., Neale, M., & Pickles, A. (1993). Genes, personality, and psychopathology: A latent class analysis of liability to symptoms of attention-deficit hyperactivity disorder in twins. In R. Plomin & G. E. McClearn (Eds.), *Nature, nurture and psychology* (pp. 285–303). Washington, DC: American Psychological Association.

Erlenmeyer-Kimling, L., & Jarvik, L. (1963). Genetics and intelligence: A review. *Science, 142,* 1477–1479.

Falconer, D. S. (1965). The inheritance of liability to certain diseases estimated from the incidence among relatives. *Annals of Human Genetics, 19,* 51–76.

Fuller, J. L., & Thompson, W. R. (1960). *Behavior genetics.* New York: Wiley.

Galton, F. (1865). Hereditary talent and character. *Macmillan's Magazine, 12,* 157–166, 318–327.

Galton, F. (1883). *Inquiries into human faculty and its development.* London: Macmillan.

Gillis, J., Gilger, J., Pennington, B., & DeFries, J. C. (1992). Attention deficit disorder in reading-disabled twins: Evidence for a genetic etiology. *Journal of Abnormal Child Psychology, 20,* 303–315.

Herrnstein, R. J. (1973). *I. Q. in the meritocracy.* Boston: Little, Brown.

Herrnstein, R. J., & Murray, C. (1994). *The bell curve: Intelligence and class structure in American life.* New York: Free Press.

Heston, L. L. (1966). Psychiatric disorders in foster home reared children of schizophrenic mothers. *British Journal of Psychiatry, 112,* 819–825.

Hetherington, E. M., & Clingempeel, W. G. (1992). Coping with marital transitions: A family systems perspective. *Monographs of the Society for Research in Child Development, 57,* Nos. 2–3, Serial No. 227.

Hetherington, E. M., Reiss, D., & Plomin, R. (Eds.). (1994). *Separate social worlds of siblings: The impact of nonshared environment on development.* Hillsdale, NJ: Erlbaum.

James, W. (1890). *Principles of psychology.* New York: Holt.

Jensen, A. R. (1969). How much can we boost IQ and scholastic achievement? *Harvard Educational Review, 39,* 1–123.

Kendler, K. S., Heath, A., Neale, M., Kessler, R., & Eaves, L. (1993). Alcoholism and major depression in women: A twin study of the causes of comorbidity. *Archives of General Psychiatry, 50,* 690–698.

Kendler, K. S., Neale, M. C., Kessler, R. C., Heath, A. C., & Eaves, L. J. (1992). Major depression and generalized anxiety disorder: Same genes, (partly) different environments? *Archives of General Psychiatry, 49,* 716–722.

Kendler, K. S., Neale, M., Kessler, R., Heath, A., & Eaves, L. (1993). Major depression and phobias: The genetic and environmental sources of comorbidity. *Psychological Medicine, 23,* 361–371.

Kevles, D. K. (1985). *In the name of eugenics: Genetics and the uses of human heredity.* New York: Knopf.

Loehlin, J. C. (1983). John Locke and behavior genetics. *Behavior Genetics, 13,* 117–121.

Lombroso, P. J., Pauls, D. L., & Leckman, J. F. (1994). Genetic mechanisms in childhood psychiatric disorders. *Journal of the American Academy of Child and Adolescent Psychiatry, 33,* 921–938.

McDougall, W. (1908). *An introduction to social psychology.* London: Methuen.

McGue, M. (1993). From proteins to cognitions: The behavioral genetics of alcoholism. In R. Plomin & G. E. McClearn (Eds.), *Nature, nurture and psychology* (pp. 245–268). Washington, DC: American Psychological Association.

McGue, M., Bouchard, T. J., Jr., Iacono, W. G., & Lykken, D. T. (1993). Behavioral genetics of cognitive ability: A life-span perspective. In R. Plomin & G. E. McClearn (Eds.), *Nature, nurture and psychology* (pp. 59–76). Washington, DC: American Psychological Association.

McGuffin, P., Owen, M. J., O'Donovan, M. C., Thapar, A., & Gottesman, I. I. (1994). *Seminars in psychiatric genetics.* London: Gaskell.

O'Connor, T. G., Hetherington, E. M., Reiss, D., & Plomin, R. (in press). A twin-sibling study of observed parent–adolescent interactions. *Child Development.*

Pike, A., McGuire, S., Hetherington, E. M., Reiss, D., & Plomin, R. (in press). Family environment and adolescent depression and antisocial behavior: A multivariate genetic analysis. *Developmental Psychology.*

Plomin, R. (1986). *Development, genetics, and psychology.* Hillsdale, NJ: Erlbaum.

Plomin, R. (1991). Genetic risk and psychosocial disorders: Links between the normal and abnormal. In M. Rutter & P. Casaer (Eds.), *Biological risk factors for psychosocial disorders* (pp. 101–138). London: Cambridge University Press.

Plomin, R. (1994a). Genetic research and identification of environmental influences: Emanuel Miller Memorial Lecture (1993). *Journal of Child Psychology and Psychiatry, 35,* 817–834.

Plomin, R. (1994b). *Genetics and experience: The interplay between nature and nurture.* Newbury Park, CA: Sage Publications.

Plomin, R. (1995). Genetics and children's experiences in the family. *Journal of Child Psychology and Psychiatry, 36,* 33–68.

Plomin, R., & Bergeman, C. S. (1991). The nature of nurture: Genetic influence on "environmental" measures. *Behavioral and Brain Sciences, 14,* 373–427.

Plomin, R., Chipuer, H. M., & Neiderhiser, J. M. (1994). Behavioral genetic evidence for the importance of nonshared environment. In E. M. Hetherington, D. Reiss, & R. Plomin (Eds.), *Separate social worlds of siblings: The impact of nonshared environment on development* (pp. 1–31). Hillsdale, NJ: Erlbaum.

Plomin, R., & Daniels, D. (1987). Why are children in the same family so different from each other? *Behavioral and Brain Sciences, 10,* 1–16.

Plomin, R., DeFries, J. C., & Loehlin, J. C. (1977). Genotype–environment interaction and correlation in the analysis of human behavior. *Psychological Bulletin, 84,* 309–322.

Plomin, R., DeFries, J. C., & McClearn, G. E. (1990). *Behavioral genetics: A primer* (2nd ed.). San Francisco: Freeman.

Plomin, R., Owen, M. J., & McGuffin, P. (1994). The genetic basis of complex human behaviors. *Science, 264,* 1733–1739.

Plomin, R., Reiss, D., Hetherington, E. M., & Howe, G. (1994). Nature and nurture: Genetic influence on measures of the family environment. *Developmental Psychology, 30,* 32–43.

Plomin, R., & Rende, R. (1991). Human behavioral genetics. *Annual Review of Psychology, 42,* 161–190.

Reiss, D., Hetherington, E. M., Plomin, R., Howe, G. W., Simmens, S. J., Henderson, S. H., O'Connor, T. J., Bussell, D. A., Anderson, E. R., & Law, T. (in press). Genetic questions for environmental studies: Differential parenting of siblings and its association with depression and antisocial behavior in adolescents. *Archives of General Psychiatry.*

Rende, R. D., Plomin, R., Reiss, D., & Hetherington, E. M. (1993). Genetic and environmental influences on depressive symptomatology in adolescence: Individual differences and extreme scores. *Journal of Child Psychology and Psychiatry, 34,* 1387–1398.

Rosenthal, D. (1970). *Genetic theory and abnormal behavior.* New York: McGraw–Hill.

Rowe, D. C. (1983a). Biometrical genetic models of self-report delinquent behavior: Twin study. *Behavior Genetics, 13,* 473–489.

Rowe, D. C. (1983b). A biometrical analysis of perceptions of family environment: A study of twin and singleton sibling kinships. *Child Development, 54,* 416–423.

Rowe, D. C. (1994). *The limits of family influence: Genes, experience, and behavior.* New York: Guilford Press.

Russell, A., & Russell, G. (1992). Child effects in socialization research: Some conceptual and data analysis issues. *Social Development, 1,* 163–184.

Rutter, M., Bailey, A., Bolton, P., & LeCouteur, A. (1993). Autism: Syndrome definition and possible genetic mechanisms. In R. Plomin & G. E. McClearn (Eds.), *Nature, nurture and psychology* (pp. 269–284). Washington, DC: American Psychological Association.

Rutter, M., Macdonald, H., Le Couteur, A., Harrington, R., Bolton, P., & Bailey, A. (1990). Genetic factors in child psychiatric disorders. II. Empirical findings. *Journal of Child Psychology and Psychiatry, 31,* 39–82.

Scarr, S. (1992). Developmental theories for the 1990s: Development and individual differences. *Child Development, 63,* 1–19.

Slater, E., & Cowie, V. (1971). *The genetics of mental disorders.* London: Oxford University Press.

Snyderman, M., & Rothman, S. (1987). Survey of expert opinion on intelligence and aptitude testing. *American Psychologist, 42,* 137–144.

Stevenson, J. (1992). Evidence for a genetic etiology in hyperactivity in children. *Behavior Genetics, 22,* 337–344.

Torrey, E. F. (1992). *Freudian fraud: The malignant effect of Freud's theory on American thought and culture.* New York: HarperCollins.

Wadsworth, S. J. (1994). School achievement. In J. C. DeFries, R. Plomin, & D. W. Fulker (Eds.), *Nature and nurture during middle childhood* (pp. 86–101). Cambridge, MA: Blackwell Publishers.

Watson, J. B. (1924). *Behaviorism.* New York: Norton.

CHAPTER 4

Blind Men and Elephants
Genetic and Other Perspectives on Schizophrenia

IRVING I. GOTTESMAN

I must apologize for invoking the timeworn but apt Indian legend of probing blind men and an elephant, each persuaded of his superior grasp of the pachyderm and the others' conceptual errors; they cannot imagine that each one of them is wrong while at the same time each one is right from their own very limited perspective. The tail is like a rope, the side is like a wall, and the leg is like a tree, but the elephant, like schizophrenia, is all of these, none of these, and much, much more. Indeed, schizophrenia may comprise more than one elephant.

Given the complexity of our common enemy—the disease or diseases called schizophrenia—different scientific techniques and disciplines undoubtedly strengthen our attempts to understand and conquer it. To achieve this goal, however, scientists of different expertise and theoretical schools, the metaphorical blind men and women, must open their eyes to the full range of data and ideas that exists.

Part I of this chapter describes the considerable evidence from one of these perspectives, genetics. Generations of blind men and women have groped and examined this part of the elephant, accumulating a very detailed

IRVING I. GOTTESMAN • Department of Psychology, University of Virginia, Charlottesville, Virginia 22903.

Genetics and Mental Illness: Evolving Issues for Research and Society, edited by Laura Lee Hall. Plenum Press, New York, 1996.

map. While it is clearly but one perspective, and an incompletely focused one at that, genetics has taught us much about schizophrenia and has more to tell.

Simply detailing the reams of data about schizophrenia that have emerged from genetic research flies in the face of what we know about this disease, what genetics has taught us. Genetics is not the whole picture. With this in mind, Part II recounts a fictional debate, adapted with minor changes from the book by Torrey, Bowler, Taylor, and Gottesman (1994), wherein scientists passionately exchange differing theoretical viewpoints of schizophrenia. In true adversarial fashion, they rally their best data and chronicle gaps and weaknesses in opposing views. Competing theories and technical approaches do not signal a mythical elephant or one that does not exist, as some critics have mistaken. Rather, the immensity of the problem and the limits of each perspective engender distinct and what sometimes seem irreconcilable views of schizophrenia. Communication of different research perspectives is a critical step toward a more complete understanding of this disease. To completely wring out an overwrought metaphor, this chapter strives to begin to open the eyes of the blind.

PART I: THE INHERITANCE OF SCHIZOPHRENIA

No educated person in 1995 can be oblivious to the fact that we are in the midst of a genetic revolution. Not only are we mapping the human genome and finding genes that lie at root of single-gene diseases and traits; we are brandishing genetic technology to better understand complex diseases, to which multiple genes and other causes contribute. But research into the causes of coronary artery disease, juvenile-onset diabetes, and the common cancers has not had to contend with the assertion that these diseases are "myths," or are "labels" used to maintain an unfair social class structure, or result from one or another kind of psychic stress traceable to how your mother raised you or how your parents communicated with each other in your presence. Although slightly caricatured, such beliefs dominated research into the major mental disorders for most of the 20th century and can still be found today with little difficulty (see Gottesman, 1994a, b; Torrey, 1995). Given the generally widespread enthusiasm for genetic and other neuroscience approaches within psychopathology today, it is difficult for the younger generation to imagine the uphill battle that has been fought for the past 45 years. Pioneers of psychiatric genetics and their students, relying on such old-fashioned strategies as interviewing and diagnosing twins, families, and adoptees, have ensured the viability of the modern psychiatric-genetic enterprise so that it can now be poised to take advantage of the methodological progress in population and molecular genetics that has blessed the study of both rare and common diseases in medical genetics (Gershon & Cloninger, 1994; King, Rotter, & Motulsky, 1992; Barnard, 1992; McGuffin et al., 1994).

Understanding the Familiality of Schizophrenia

As there may be lingering doubts about the established familiality of schizophrenia and, further, that the familiality is largely under genetic control rather than arising largely from shared experiences, a brief recapitulation may be in order. Table 1 shows the results of pooling more than 40 systematic family and twin studies conducted between 1920 and 1991 (see Gottesman, 1991) that took place in Western Europe. While diagnostic standards varied, ranging from Kraepelinian to Bleulerian, studies using subjects with syndromes secondary to likely organic causes (phenocopies) involving alcohol or head injuries (see Davison, 1992; Saugstad & Odegaard, 1986) have been screened out. Criticisms of such studies on the grounds that they did not use the currently fashionable as well as reliable structured interviews do not stand up to scrutiny as recent studies using such instruments yield very similar results (e.g., Kendler et al., 1993; Maier et al., 1993).

Table 1

Risks of Schizophrenia (Definite plus Probable) for Relatives of Schizophrenics[a]

Relationship	Morbid risk (%)
General population	1%
Spouses of patients	2%
Third-degree relatives	
First cousins	2%
Second-degree relatives	
Uncles/aunts	2%
Nephews/nieces	4%
Grandchildren	5%
Half siblings	6%
First-degree relatives	
Parents	6%
Siblings	9%
Children	13%
Siblings with one schizophrenic parent	17%
DZ twins	16%
MZ twins	48%

[a]Adapted from Gottesman, I. I. (1991). *Schizophrenic genesis: The origins of madness*. San Francisco: Freeman.

These data can only be evaluated against the background fact that the lifetime risk or probability of a random member of the population developing a case of schizophrenia is close to 1 in 100 or 1% (Jablensky, 1993; but see Torrey, 1989, and Stromgren, 1987). Kendler *et al.* (1993), working only with DSM-IIIR-defined schizophrenia in rural Ireland and using structured interviews, found that 2.6% of parents and 10.1% of siblings also met these criteria for schizophrenia; the comparable general population morbid risk using the same operationalized criteria was 0.5% (rather than the typical 1.0%). When schizoaffective disorders—mainly schizophrenia and other nonaffective psychoses—were counted as "affected," the risk to the combined sample of parents and siblings went up to 12.9%, approximating the risks in the classical studies in Table 1. A rationale for broadening the range of phenotypes that provide valid information about the schizophrenia genotype will be illustrated below. In other words, existing disorders emanate from genes and other factors.

It is no longer necessary to spend time defending the pre-World War II-initiated twin studies of schizophrenia as we have six modern studies in the literature and a preliminary report on a seventh ongoing in Nagasaki, Japan (Tsujita *et al.,* 1992). Table 2 presents the probandwise rates (McGue, 1992; Torrey, 1992) without age correction for the six studies using somewhat varied but reasonable definitions of schizophrenia. By applying various contemporary operational criteria for making the diagnosis of schizophrenia to the United Kingdom study (Gottesman & Shields, 1972), Farmer *et al.* (1987) and McGuffin *et al.* (1993) demonstrated that the original results, which depended on experienced clinical judges, remained intact. The median identical twin concordance rate of 46% and the same-sex fraternal twin rate of 14% for the six studies are reasonably close to the prewar studies with all of their alleged flaws once allowance is made for differences in severity of illness. The newer Norwegian study (Onstad *et al.,* 1991) meets most of the objections leveled at twin studies by using structured interviews with a national sample and by using DSM-IIIR criteria; it is gratifying to see that the results are a close match to the other studies in Table 2 where the twin samples were also personally interviewed. It needs to be noted that the senior Norwegian coinvestigator, Einar Kringlen, is well-known for his skepticism about overly genetic explanations. The preliminary probandwise rates for DSM-IIIR schizophrenia in the Nagasaki work is 53% in 17 MZ pairs and 0% in six same-sex DZ pairs; these rates go up to 57 and 33% when the diagnoses studied include schizophreniform (resembling schizophrenia proper but with a duration of symptoms less than 6 months) and schizotypal disorders (a personality disorder with attenuated features of schizophrenia other than delusions and hallucinations) in probands and in cotwins.

Table 2
Concordance Rates for Schizophrenia in Newer Twin Studies[a]

	MZ pairs		DZ pairs	
	Total pairs	Probandwise rate (%)	Total pairs	Probandwise rate (%)
Finland, 1963/1971	17	35	20	13
Norway, 1967	55	45	90	15
Denmark, 1973	21	56	41	27
United Kingdom, 1966/1987	22	58	33	15
Norway, 1991	31	48	28	4
United States, 1969/1983	164	31	268	6
Pooled concordance (excluding USA)				
Median	146	48	212	15
Weighted mean		48		16
Pooled concordance (all studies)				
Median	310	46	480	14
Weighted mean		39		10

[a]Adapted from Gottesman, I. I. (1991). *Schizophrenia genesis: The origins of madness.* San Francisco: Freeman.

Roles for Experience in the Liability to Schizophrenia

Clearly, from Tables 1 and 2, schizophrenia is familial but that is not enough from which to infer the relative roles of genes and of environment, be it pre-, peri-, and postnatal, in the etiology of the disorder. Psychodynamically oriented theorists would use these observations to implicate one or another dysfunctional aspect of shared environments or experiences, while genetically oriented theorists would use the very same observations to confirm their beliefs that schizophrenia "ran in families" because genes ran in families. Both sides are each partially correct but there are constraints on etiological speculations. The disorder does not appear to be transmitted as an infectious disease among adults in the majority of cases or by psychological "contagion" because the spouses and inpatient ward personnel have quite low risks. In addition, half siblings of people with schizophrenia, although having the same environmental exposures as full siblings, have risks that better match their degree of gene sharing. It is theoretically possible, however, that transmission of the infectious agent could occur during the intrauterine period of development or in early childhood. The fields of immunology and virology are new to the schizophrenia scene with rapidly changing results, often difficult to replicate because of a shortage of specialists. Crow (1994), in an editorial, reviews the evidence for the role of prenatal exposure to influenza as a significant cause of schizophrenia and sees inconsistencies and contradictions worth noting by subsequent researchers. Just recently, using cerebrospinal fluid and blood from just nine sets of our twins discordant for schizophrenia, Sierra-Honigmann, Carbone, and Yolken (1995) found that no virus-specific nucleic acids could be implicated [cytomegalovirus, HIV, influenza A, Borna disease virus, and bovine viral (BDVD)] for a persistent or latent infection caused by these viruses. Other viruses, and there are many, may be implicated in further research (Torrey, 1991).

Adoption strategies are needed to gain perspective on the role of some of the possible causes of schizophrenia. Only one of these important contributions will be discussed here (see Heston, 1966; Tienari et al., 1994). The final results from the Danish national sample of adoptees, begun by Seymour Kety and colleagues in the 1960s, in which the adoptees who grew up to develop schizophrenia and their biological and adoptive relatives, are now available (Kety et al., 1994). Kendler, Gruenberg, and Kinney (1994) applied DSM-III criteria to the index and control adoptees, to their biological relatives to whom they had had no exposure, and to the adoptive relatives who had reared, or been reared with, the adoptees. Neither group of adoptive relatives had an above-baseline level of schizophrenia spectrum disorders (1–2%). The schizophrenia spectrum adoptees, however, defined to include not only schizophrenia but also schizoaffective disorder-mainly schizophrenic and schizotypal personality (and paranoid personality in the relatives), had a prevalence of the same disorders of 23.5% among the interviewed first-degree relatives, contrasted with a prevalence of 4.7% among biological relatives of normal control adoptees. Such a definitive outcome confirms the essentially same findings with smaller samples in the literature using adoption strategies (McGuffin et al., 1994) and nullifies strong postnatal environmental (e.g., bad relationships) hypotheses about the transmission of schizophrenia.

Given the evidence in Tables 1 and 2 and the new Danish and Finnish adoption results, it is too easy to lose perspective on the essential role that must be preserved for the contribution of environmental factors, be they biological or psychosocial. Recall that the concordance rate in identical twins is so far from 100% as to compel attention to nongenetic contributions to the liability to developing schizophrenia; indeed, it laid the foundation for our research on discordant identical twins reported below (Torrey et al., 1994). The ingredients that characterize such influences deserve close attention and empirical research (Day, 1986; Tienari et al., 1994; Warner, 1994).

A Multifactorial Oligogenic Threshold Model Resolution

Sing and Moll (1990) have provided a master strategic plan for unraveling the genetic basis of schizophrenia and other major mental disorders, but they did so while talking about coronary artery disease (CAD). In this instance, imitation is not only flattering but essential as the problems encountered in the unraveling are so analogous. Researchers in psychiatric genetics can only envy and try to emulate the advanced stages of the plan as it has been applied so far in CAD. A choice among genetic models for explaining the intergenerational transmission of schizophrenia is available and outlined in Table 3 (see Moldin & Gottesman, 1995; Prescott & Gottesman, 1993; Gottesman & McGue, 1991). Each of the six models may be partially correct as they appear to be for CAD, but the weighting to be given each model in a market-basket explanation of causes for the phenotypes is a matter of great debate, as will be shortly evident. The merits of multifactorial and mixed models became apparent through data analyses and computer simulations. Enthusiasm for such models had been kindled some 30 years ago by discussions with Falconer (Gottesman & Shields, 1967) and with Odegaard (1952, 1972). Without slowing for details here, we conducted extensive model fitting with the family and twin data summarized earlier. A single major locus (SML) even allowing for varying penetrances could be rejected for the data as a whole. One gene alone producing schizophrenia is not consistent with the data. We next shifted to a mixed model approach and ran 275 combinations of various degrees of penetrance for a putative major gene, various degrees of heritability, and various proportions of phenocopies (people with schizophrenia without a copy of the major gene). We already had shown that the combined data were consistent with a

Table 3
Six Models of Genetic Transmission of Schizophrenia

	Sources of familial resemblance		
Genetic model	Major locus	Polygenes	Common environment
Single major locus	Yes	No	No
With intra-allelic heterogeneity	Yes	No	No
With interlocus heterogeneity	>1	No	No
Mixed model	Yes	Yes	Yes
Multifactorial oligogenic	>1	Yes	Yes
Multifactorial polygenic	No	Yes	Yes

multifactorial threshold model with high heritability, that is, a standard model for non-Mendelian disorders wherein a genetic predisposition (unspecified) plus environmental factors (unspecified) pushes one over a threshold into an episode of schizophrenia. The new simulations added two further models consistent with the observed risks in the different classes of relatives. A mixed model with a major gene with penetrance > 0.40, but with a very high proportion of phenocopies (> 0.60), a large residual heritability > 0.60, and, frustrating the would-be linkage analyst, a low gene frequency of 0.003 was consistent with the data.

This would mean that most people with schizophrenia do not have the major gene but are affected because of their high multifactorial loading. The other consistent mixed model had a major gene with low penetrance, < 0.20, a high residual heritability > 0.60, and it was not sensitive to the proportion of phenocopies. With this latter model, most people with schizophrenia will have the gene. But its low penetrance will make it unwieldy for the usual linkage approaches, as most people with the gene will not have the disease.

With these simulations in hand, we sought to answer two questions: How often would the models, if true, result in families with multiple cases of schizophrenia? And, to what extent would researchers be able to isolate multigenerational, multiply-affected families with a major gene for schizophrenia? Our use of 50,000 simulated families for each of the four consistent models, allowing for expected marriage rates (Gottesman, 1991) and expected sibship sizes, resulted in paradoxical and disquieting findings. Only 2 families in 200,000 contained five or more affected members and only 11 families in 200,000 contained four or more affected members! Multiplex ascertainment for one of the consistent mixed models did result in most sampled families carrying the major gene, but the penetrance was only 0.10 and the model generated a high-false-positive rate with 52% of normals having the gene but not having the schizophrenia phenotype. Consider these simulation studies to be cost-effective "thought experiments" that may guide further empirical research.

Single major locus forms of schizophrenia probably exist, but the simulations suggest that such forms are likely to result either from a highly prevalent gene with a very low penetrance or from a highly penetrant gene with a very low gene frequency. A useful and sobering analogy to Huntington's disease illustrates the need for more than a single major locus model (Table 4). Approximately 20% of people with Huntington's disease in the literature (for the first two-thirds of the century) presented with enough schizophrenia symptoms to receive what is a false diagnosis of paranoid schizophrenia. Given the lifetime risk for Huntington's disease

Table 4
Schizophrenia and Schizophrenia-like Psychosis in Offspring of Schizophrenic Twins[a]

	Index parents			
	Monozygotic		Dizygotic	
	Schizophrenic twins ($n = 11$)	"Normal" cotwins ($n = 6$)	Schizophrenic twins ($n = 10$)	"Normal" cotwins ($n = 20$)
Number of offspring	47	24	27	52
Schizophrenia and schizophrenia-like	6	4	4	1
Morbid risk	16.8%	17.4%	17.4%	2.1%

[a]Gottesman, I. I., and Bertelsen, A. (1989). Confirming unexpressed genotypes for schizophrenia. Risks in the offspring of Fischer's Danish identical and fraternal discordant twins. *Archives of General Psychiatry* 46, 867–872.

of 5 per 100,000 and, for example, the lifetime risk for clinical schizophrenia in a total population in southern Sweden (Essen-Moller *et al.*, 1956) of 139 per 10,000, we can determine the proportion of schizophrenia-like psychoses actually caused by this dominant gene, now mapped to 4p16.3 (HDCRG, 1993). The arithmetic reveals that 7 of every 10,000 people with schizophrenia would have this major gene, leaving, of course, the remaining 9993 cases for other causes. Similarly, other genes at other loci could, in principle, be identified by studying those few multiplex families that exist with appropriate probes and standard linkage analyses. Each such discovery would be important to the whole enterprise of accounting for as many phenotypes as possible and could, in principle, help to specify some aspects of the neurochemistry and other factors in the path between the phenotype and the genes that would generalize to the more common varieties with more complex etiologies.

A speculative combined or "ecumenical" model for the etiologies of schizophrenia, informed by the work reviewed so far, makes provision for slow viruses as sufficient and/or as triggers for vulnerable genotypes; for other primarily environmental causes including those secondary to drug intoxications (dopamine agonists) or brain lesions; for rare single-locus causes; and some proportion of each of the kinds of mixed and multifactorial genetic models. The strategies outlined by Sing and Moll for CAD and the results of family and twin studies of CAD at both the clinical and molecular levels (e.g., Berg, 1990; Motulsky & Brunzell, 1992; Burke & Motulsky, 1992; Devereux & Brown, 1992) are compatible with such ecumenicism.

Some Further Complications

The study of twins, both concordant and discordant for clinical schizo-phrenia, has made important contributions to the specification of the pheno-types and the endophenotypes (a term to demark steps in the causal chain that intervene between the gene and the phenotype such as variations in neurochemistry or in dopamine receptor number) (Gottesman & Shields, 1972) that could be "scored" as relevant to unmasking the schizophrenia genotype(s). However, the necessary genotype may remain completely un-expressed as evidenced by the study of the offspring of MZ twins discordant for schizophrenia. Gottesman and Bertelsen (1989) reported on the adult offspring of 21 identical twins [monozygotic twins (MZ)] and 41 fraternal twin [dizygotic (DZ)] pairs studied earlier by Fischer (1971) where the twins had been born between 1870 and 1920 and their offspring were followed up to 1985. The risk among the adult children of both the MZ and DZ probands with schizophrenia was 17% as might have been expected. The risk of schizophrenia among the 24 offspring of phenotypically normal MZ cotwins was also 17%, while it was only 2% among the offspring of the phenotypically normal DZ cotwins. Such a finding suggests that the normal MZ cotwins carried and transmitted the relevant genotype, without expressing it themselves. The cotwins were not scrutinized with "star wars" technology, just interviews or a clean bill of health in various national Danish registers (psychiatric, criminal, death); the results need to be repli-cated. The only other attempt to use such a strategy was reported in Norway by Kringlen and Cramer (1989) using younger MZ twins. Five of twenty-eight (18%) offspring of twins with schizophrenia had schizophrenia spec-trum disorders as did only 2 of 45 (4%) offspring of the unaffected cotwins; with these sample sizes the rates were not different statistically. They are, however, consistent with the Danish findings which were significantly higher than the rate in normal DZ cotwin offspring. Further follow-up of the Norwegian sample when they are further through the risk period for devel-oping schizophrenia will add important information. Both studies support the idea that discordant pairs do not necessarily represent nongenetic, environmentally caused phenocopies and that false negatives in the pedi-grees used for linkage analyses are to be expected to confound the results.

Clearly, "normality" can hide the presence of a relevant genotype for schizophrenia. But what kinds of psychopathology can emerge from "schizophrenia genes"? That is, what characterizes the clinical spectrum of liability to schizophrenia (Claridge, 1994; Moldin et al., 1990; Prescott & Gottesman, 1993)? Only a partial answer can be provided here (see Lenzenweger, 1993; Iacono & Clementz, 1993; Kendler & Diehl, 1993). The consensus from recent family, twin, and adoption efforts to specify schizophrenia-relevant spectrum disorders implicates schizotypal personality, schizoaffective psychoses-mainly schizophrenic, atypical and schizophreniform psychoses, affective psychoses with mood-incongruent delusions, and, probably, schizoid and paranoid personality disorders. Delusional disorder is too rare to generate stable findings. Some of the implicated conditions may only be indicators within the biological families of known schizophrenic probands and will not have specificity when encountered in the general population. The specificity of schizophrenia-spectrum disorders, however, lends no support to efforts to revitalize the old notion of *Einheitspsychosen*—a 19th century idea that there was a "unitary" psychosis with no distinction possible between schizophrenia and manic-depression (Crow, 1990; Stromgren, 1995).

In the brief span of years since 1988 when positive linkage was reported between schizophrenia and a DNA marker on the long arm of chromosome number 5, a growth industry has been spawned in the field of psychiatric genetics with the production of negative and nonreplicated linkage and association results for both random markers and reasonable candidate genes for various dopamine neurotransmitter receptors and transporters (for reviews see Coon *et al.,* 1994; Kendler & Diehl, 1993; McGuffin *et al.,* 1994). The good news buried in such an outcome is that the details of an exclusion map are being filled in at a good rate. Owen (1992) has asked whether schizophrenia will become a "graveyard for molecular geneticists?" to remind us of an earlier sentiment expressed about the role of neuropathologists in schizophrenia research. Fortunately for us, he answers his own rhetorical question by concluding that "talk of graveyards is premature" and that the "application of molecular genetics to the study of schizophrenia is still in its infancy" (p. 292). Note also that neuropathology in schizophrenia has been resuscitated both by the introduction of brain imaging (Andreasen, 1989) and by a neurodevelopmental orientation (Mednick, 1995; Walker, 1994; Weinberger, 1987; and "Dr. D'Velupmoni" below).

Absent definitive knowledge about the pathophysiology of schizophrenia (Torrey, 1991), we lack such candidate genes as those associated with the apolipoproteins and other lipid-related genes in CAD (Berg *et al.,* 1990). However, the dopamine theory of schizophrenia (see Mendlewicz and Hippius, 1992) stemming from the successful pharmacological treatments of the symptoms of schizophrenia has given rise to linkage and association studies with a family of candidate genes for D1, D2, D3, D4, and D5 receptors with disappointingly negative results (e.g., Coon *et al.,* 1993, 1994). A novel, "bottom-up" association approach has recently been suggested by Sobell, Heston, and Sommer (1993) that examines neurotransmission candidate genes for any DNA sequence variation that might affect protein structure or the level of gene expression (see Berg, 1990, on level and variability genes in CAD). Once identified, the prevalence of sequence variations is determined in a model panel of unrelated people with schizophrenia and in their normal controls to hunt for association. Two common mutations in the PAH gene that causes phenylketonuria (PKU)—PKU patients sometimes have symptoms of schizophrenia—were screened in this fashion with negative results.

Do not despair. Almost none of the studies in the literature have used an informed definition of the relevant phenotypes as described above. Furthermore, many candidate genes remain to be tested both for linkage and for association. Regulatory pathways involving neurotransmission remain a target of opportunity in addition to receptors as do the genes involved in transportation of transmitters. The major inhibitory neurotransmitter in brain is GABA and it alone has several thousand possible receptor subtypes (Barnard, 1992). As Owen noted, the field is still in its infancy. There is no need to choose between a top-down and a bottom-up strategy in researching the etiologies of schizophrenia as there is a need for both reductionism and neo-Darwinism to solve the problems outlined above.

PART II: COMPETING VIEWS OF SCHIZOPHRENIA

In an effort to shed light on the pathophysiology of schizophrenia and useful endophenotypes a new study of identical twins discordant for schizophrenia was initiated (Torrey *et al.*, 1994) at the Twin Study Unit at St. Elizabeths Hospital, Washington, DC. Small control groups of MZ twins concordant for schizophrenia, discordant for bipolar disorder, and concordant for normality were also recruited. Virological, genetic, and neurodevelopmental hypotheses were pursued with a range of devices including metabolic and imaging probes (e.g., MRI, rCBF, PET, SPECT), interviews, eye-tracking, fingerprints to sample prenatal growth, and personality tests.

I present here, with minor changes from Torrey *et al.* (1994), a "bare bones" summary of the initial findings from the study as a prelude to a spirited debate among "fictional" researchers who hold differing, but reconcilable, views about the weight to give to different, partially correct views both about the origins of schizophrenia and about the factors that influence its course and outcome in individual sufferers.

1. The research project described in detail in Torrey *et al.* (1994) included 66 pairs of identical twins studied over a 6-year period: 27 pairs discordant for schizophrenia; 13 pairs concordant for schizophrenia; 8 pairs discordant for bipolar disorder; 8 pairs

within normal limits; 8 pairs with "mixed" diagnoses; and 2 pairs not fully testable.

2. A family history of serious mental disorder was found among both the concordant and the discordant twin pairs (15 and 26% of their families).

3. Pregnancy and birth abnormalities appeared to be important in the etiology of at least 30% of the twins with schizophrenia.

4. About 30% of the twins who developed schizophrenia had been different from their nonschizophrenic cotwin before entering school in their behavior, cognition, or neurological intactness; many appeared to have noticeable central nervous system dysfunction (termed "pandysmaturation" by Dr. Barbara Fish).

5. The role of head trauma or childhood physical illnesses in schizophrenia could not be answered by our data.

6. Intriguing but preliminary viral research implicated a link between pestiviruses and schizophrenia in 10 of 25 tested pairs of discordant identical twins.

7. Changes in brain structure were prominent in the MRIs (magnetic resonance images) in the twins with schizophrenia. For example, the affected twin had a smaller right hippocampus–amygdala region 81% of the time and a smaller left region 78% of the time, compared to the well cotwin.

8. Although changes in brain structure did not correlate with severity of schizophrenia, ventricular enlargements were associated with lower birth weight and early age of divergence from cotwin.

9. Changes in brain function measured by cerebral blood flow (hypofrontality), neurological tests, and eye-tracking dysfunction were prominent in affected twins.

10. Twins concordant for schizophrenia did not differ clinically or in presumed etiological factors from twins with schizophrenia in discordant pairs.

11. Despite the information available on brain structure and function, it is not yet possible to use such measures diagnostically to predict whether any given individual is or will in the future develop schizophrenia (Bertelsen and Gottesman, 1990).

A Crossfire-like Debate to Prepare the Way for Further Research Progress

We have assembled three fictional authorities. "Dr. Mendel M. Malgene" represents the genetic viewpoint, "Dr. Dena S. Daverus" takes the virological position, and "Dr. A. Dominic D'Velupmoni" speaks from a neurodevelopmental perspective. Each was asked to summarize the important findings from the study and then to critique each other's summaries.

Geneticist's Viewpoint: Dr. Malgene. I have the dubious honor of leading off the discussion today and exposing my genetic bias before I have had the opportunity to hear from my colleagues. I think it is important to note at the outset that this research project was not planned to answer genetic questions. On the contrary, it explicitly focused its primary attention on monozygotic twins in which one is affected with schizophrenia or bipolar disorder and the other is well. As such, this project selectively focused on individuals who are *least* likely to have genetic variants of these diseases, thereby maximizing the opportunity to observe and to identify environmental and experiential contributors to the causes and courses of schizophrenia. Many identical twins in which only one is affected may represent phenocopies of the true disease; that is, they have the outward manifestations and symptoms but not the underlying genetic substrate. We accept that some cases of schizophrenia and bipolar disorder are not genetic in origin, and this project focused on that hypothetical group.

Regarding the paucity of family history for schizophrenia or other serious mental diseases among the twins discordant (and especially those concordant) for schizophrenia, one likely reason for this is that the researchers did not look hard enough. Recall that in the earliest stages of the project they collected personality questionnaires (MMPIs) on first-degree relatives (mother, father, brothers, and sisters) of their subjects, but then the researchers abandoned this procedure because they found it to be too intrusive. That was a mistake, for if they had continued with the MMPIs, they almost certainly would have found more members of the families, especially the families of the concordant pairs, to have schizoid personality disorder and other diagnoses considered to be part of the schizophrenia spectrum. For example, in reviewing older twin studies, Cadoret found among the families of the twins "a high proportion of individuals with significant character abnormalities or neurotic symptoms" (Cadoret, 1973; Gottesman, 1987). Kringlen also found more family history of serious mental diseases in his twin study than were found in the present study. The researchers should have personally interviewed all first-degree relatives, and in this way they could have truly ascertained the prevalence of serious mental illnesses among the relatives.

In this regard, I would like to bring to my colleagues' attention the important findings of Gottesman and Bertelsen, who found an increased risk (17%) of schizophrenia among the children of the *well* twins in Fischer's Danish study of identical twins discordant for schizophrenia (Gottesman &

Bertelsen, 1989) (Table 4). This would appear to be strong evidence suggesting that the well twins in the present study may also be carrying a schizophrenia gene that, for one reason or another, is not being expressed. We know also that genes may be pleiotropic, by which I mean that the same gene may be expressed in a variety of ways in different individuals. For example, the dominant gene known to cause neurofibromatosis [a misdiagnosis of Mr. Merrick the Elephant Man] may express itself variously as tan spots on the skin, areas of skin depigmentation, abnormalities of the bones, or as tumors of the nerves. If a single gene can express itself in so many different ways, then why should we be surprised if the gene or genes implicated in schizophrenia also manifest themselves in a variety of ways in different individuals?

Within the present study there is some evidence that the well cotwins in the discordant pairs may have some genetic loading for the disease. Note that the discordant twins with a family history of serious mental diseases have higher scores for minor physical anomalies; a logical explanation for this association is that one or more genes are responsible for both phenomena. There is also a trend for the affected twins with a family history of serious mental diseases to have an earlier age of divergence, which also suggests a genetic subgroup.

Several additional findings support my belief that at least some of the cotwins in this project are carriers of the disease. The concordant twins have significantly fewer obstetrical complications than the discordant twins, which would be consistent with the concordant twins having a more genetic form of the disease. Also note that the well cotwins in the discordant pairs had scores for neurological abnormalities that fell midway between the scores of the twins with schizophrenia and the normal controls. The well cotwins in the discordant pairs also had more abnormalities on neuropsychological tests than did the normal controls.

I would caution my colleagues about interpreting the genetic aspects of schizophrenia too narrowly. We are just beginning to learn how complex genetic makeup can be (Gottesman, 1994a,b). Not only do we have proposed single-gene and polygenic models for schizophrenia, but the genes involved may also be scattered at different sites on the same chromosome or on different chromosomes. Some researchers have postulated that there are both major genes and minor genes involved. The genes may also have varying levels of penetrance, by which I mean that they may be expressed more overtly in one individual but more covertly in another.

Furthermore, the gene or genes involved in schizophrenia may do so in one of many ways. The schizophrenia gene(s) may be like the gene that causes phenylketonuria, a metabolic disease that begins in childhood, in which the gene causes a defect in the enzyme that normally breaks down phenylalanine; the symptoms of the disease come from the accumulation of phenylalanine in the brain. The child does not get phenylketonuria unless phenylalanine is ingested in the diet. This is an example of a genetic disease that only becomes manifest if certain environmental conditions are present.

Alternatively, the schizophrenia gene(s) may act by altering the metabolism of dopamine and its metabolites. In one sense, the dopamine theory of schizophrenia can be considered a subtype of the genetic theory. Recently there has been speculation that multiple sclerosis may be caused by genetically transmitted defects in myelin basic protein (Tienari *et al.,* 1992), and schizophrenia may be caused in a similar fashion. Since genes govern the embryological developmental processes of the brain and its susceptibility to decreased oxygen or other environmental insults, developmental theories may also be considered as a kind of genetic theory. Furthermore, genes are known to play an important role in determining susceptibility of the body to various infectious agents, and it is well known that the body's response to specific bacteria and viruses is partly determined by genetics. In that sense, the viral theory of schizophrenia is also a type of genetic theory.

Finally, I would add that recent research on adoptees and on identical twins raised apart has strongly supported the importance of genetics in determining normal personality traits. Since genes play such a prominent role in normal personality traits, it is certainly reasonable to expect that they also play a prominent role in determining the abnormal personality traits we categorize as schizophrenia.

Virologist's Viewpoint: Dr. Daverus. In reviewing the findings from this ambitious study, I was impressed by how well the findings fit a viral hypothesis of schizophrenia. Of course, the report of finding antibodies to pestiviruses in the plasma and cerebrospinal fluid of some affected twins is exciting, but that is only a preliminary report and needs to be replicated. Additional findings of interest include the increased number of spontaneous abortions among the mothers of the discordant twins, and the trend toward a winter–spring birth seasonality in the discordant twins who have more perinatal indicators of risk. Both of these could be explained by prenatal viral infections.

What I am most impressed with is the evidence that the schizophrenia disease process goes back to the period prior to birth in some cases, and perhaps to the first few weeks after birth in others. The cumulative evidence from minor physical anomalies, total finger ridge counts, and obstetrical complications is impressive in confirming that something begins to go wrong in the early developmental stages of life in some cases of schizophrenia, even though the individual does not develop the actual symptoms of the disease until many years later.

Recent studies have shown how frequently viruses may be transmitted from mother to fetus across the placenta or during the birth process. For example, hepatitis C virus, which is in the same Flavivirus family as pestiviruses, is commonly transmitted from infected mothers to fetuses and then initiates a silent disease process or chronic carrier state (Thaler *et al.,* 1991). Recent studies have shown that the HIV virus is commonly transmitted from infected mothers to their children late in pregnancy or at the time of delivery (Ehrnst *et al.,* 1991). Similarly, one-third of babies born to women who have a primary herpes simplex virus genital infection will become infected during the birth process (Brown *et al.,* 1991). We now know that many different viruses are capable of getting into the brain and remaining latent there for many years before causing symptomatic infection. And we know that viruses may infect only one twin *in utero* in an identical twin pair (reviewed in Torrey *et al.,* 1994).

Even following birth, we know that both twins in an identical pair may be infected with a virus and yet have very different reactions to that virus. In one case reported, identical twins both had measles at age 4; 10 years later one of them developed subacute sclerosing panencephalitis, a severe and ultimately fatal complication of measles infection, but the other twin did not (Whitaker, Sever, & Engel, 1972). In another case, both twins were infected with the hepatitis B virus; one of them developed active disease, but the other only developed a chronic carrier state (Peters, Reeves, & Purcell, 1977).

The consistent finding of smaller hippocampus–amygdala complexes in the affected twins is also intriguing. Something either has impaired the development of that part of the brain or has caused cell death to reduce its size. There are a limited number of agents that could reduce the size of the hippocampus–amygdala, and a viral infection is one of them. We now know that you would not necessarily find neuropathological changes if a viral infection were responsible for the brain changes. Early in development the fetus's immune system is not sufficiently developed to mount an immune response to the infection. And later in development it has been shown that viruses can sometimes disrupt cell function—for example, alter the production of dopamine or another neurotransmitter—without producing any cellular pathology visible under a microscope (Oldstone *et al.,* 1982).

I also agree with Dr. Malgene's comments regarding the importance of genetic predisposition to viral diseases. We know there is a genetic factor that plays a role in determining whether any given virus will infect the brain, and this genetic factor has been shown to affect viruses that are in the same family as the pestivirus (Roos, 1985). Recall also that for the poliovirus, a virus that has been carefully studied in the central nervous system, the pairwise concordance rate for infection in identical twins is 36%

and in fraternal twins 6%; these concordance rates are virtually identical to those for schizophrenia.

Finally, I would like to remind my colleagues that viral infections that might cause schizophrenia may also begin after the perinatal period. I was especially impressed by the history of discordant pair DS-19, in which neurological ("a strange gait") and behavioral problems began at age 5, with no preexisting indicators of risk or illness. Discordant pair DS-25, in which the schizophrenia began immediately following a viral illness and rash, and pair DS-3, in which symptoms began shortly after a severe flulike syndrome, are also noteworthy.

Developmentalist's Viewpoint: Dr. D'Velupmoni. I have the pleasure of going last, which is appropriate because my explanation for the causes of schizophrenia both builds on and incorporates the explanations of my colleagues. It seems to me that this twin study provides strong evidence for a developmental theory of the disease, one substantially more complex than a genetic or viral explanation alone. I am reminded of a quotation by Dr. R. S. Nowakowski who, in a review of brain development, said: "The human central nervous system is, without a doubt, the single most complicated organ in the body, and the processes involved in its development are commensurately complex" (Nowakowski, 1987).

Perhaps the most striking finding from this exhaustive study is that no single etiological factor is prominent. There are indications that *something* is going on in the developing brain of some of the people who later develop schizophrenia, but no one factor appears to be clearly associated. The pathology observed on the MRIs includes some dilatation of the cerebral ventricles, as well as some loss of volume of the hippocampus–amygdala complex. Both of these changes are nonspecific and, at least the latter, most likely take place during early stages of brain development.

The combination of nonspecific indicators of developmental problems and nonspecific cerebral pathology suggests a nonspecific or multietiological developmental explanation. The developmental theory postulates that any one of a number of etiological agents could initiate the causative cascade leading to schizophrenia *if* that agent affected the brain at a crucial stage of development. The etiological agents could include, in the words of Dr. Daniel R. Weinberger, "a hereditary encephalopathy or predilection to environmental injury, an infection or postinfectious state, damage from an immunologic disorder, perinatal trauma or encephalopathy, toxin exposure early in development, a primary metabolic disease, or other early developmental events" (Weinberger, 1987).

Once the original insult takes place at a critical stage of brain development, the damage is done. In most cases, however, its effects are not immediately noticeable, except perhaps for nonspecific signs such as lack of coordination or behavioral problems in childhood. In the majority of cases, the effects of the early brain damage must await the maturation of the brain, at which point the developmental damage becomes noticeable as the signs and symptoms of schizophrenia. There are now rat models that show you can cause lesions in the hippocampus of a rat's brain during early development, but the effects of the lesions will not show up behaviorally until the rat matures (Lipska, Jaskiw, & Weinberger, 1993). Some people believe that this developmental model also explains many cases of epilepsy as well as schizophrenia.

There is one other finding from this study that is important from a developmental point of view. The affected twins who scored the highest on indicators of perinatal liability, such as minor physical anomalies, total finger ridge counts, obstetrical complications, and lower birth weight, tended to do *better* clinically than the affected twins with fewer indicators of perinatal liability. Most theories of schizophrenia would postulate that these affected twins should do *worse* than the others because the brain damage occurred at an earlier state or was more extensive. The developmental theory, however, might explain this by postulating that the earlier damage allowed for the formation of alternative pathways of neural development, thus partially compensating for the injury.

In deference to Dr. Malgene, I should add that the developmental theory does not ignore genetics. Brain development is largely under genetic control, and it would be reasonable to expect that some individuals would have a higher degree of genetic predisposition to brain insults. The genes might operate directly to cause abnormal migration of cells or abnormal innervation of a particular area of the brain, or the genes might operate indirectly by making the hippocampus more susceptible to decreased oxygen or other insults.

Discussion. The participants were encouraged to critique each other's presentation, restricting their remarks to the twin study as much as possible; poetic licenses were issued.

Dr. Daverus: Let me begin by raising questions about Dr. Malgene's presentation. I would first note that most of his presentation focused on theoretical genetic models of disease rather than on this twin study *per se*. The reason he did this, I believe, is that the present twin study produced very little support for genetic theories. The concordant twins compared to the discordant twins did not have a higher frequency of family history of serious mental illness as one would expect in a genetically transmitted disease. This finding is in agreement with the study by Gottesman and Shields (1972) in which the concordant twins compared to the discordant twins also did not have a greater family history of serious mental diseases.

One would also expect the concordant twins, in whom genetic factors by definition are maximal, to differ from the affected discordant twins, in whom genetic factors are presumed to be less important. When the two groups were compared, however, they were remarkably alike in clinical manifestations, including negative symptoms, neurological abnormalities, and neuropsychological functioning, as well as in indicators of perinatal liability such as minor physical anomalies, total finger ridge counts, and obstetrical complications.

Perhaps even more important is the fact that the twins who do have a family history of serious mental illnesses do not appear to be significantly different from the twins with no such history. On both clinical measures and etiological indicators, the two groups are alike. There were also no significant differences between the groups on brain structure as measured by MRIs. No single measure emerged as a possible genetic marker for schizophrenia. Even eye-tracking dysfunction, which has been widely considered to be a genetic marker for this disease, was not consistently found in the well cotwins in the discordant pairs, thereby casting doubt on its candidacy as a genetic marker.

DR. D'VELUPMONI: I would also like to question some of Dr. Malgene's statements. He said that evidence of psychopathology was not found in the well cotwins in the discordant pairs because the researchers did not look closely enough. We must be cautious in making such statements. One of the things we should have learned from the psychiatric misadventures with Freudian theory is that one can find psychopathology, loosely defined, in virtually everybody if one looks closely enough. The question is not whether there is any psychopathology in the well cotwins, but rather whether there is any *more* psychopathology in these cotwins than could be found in any group of identical twins randomly selected off the street.

Dr. Malgene does a nice job of reviewing genetic models for phenylketonuria, neurofibromatosis, and other disorders. The important question, however, is not whether such models *can* theoretically account for the findings in schizophrenia, but rather how well such models actually fit the findings. I believe we all accept the fact that genes play *some* role in the etiology of schizophrenia, but postulating that schizophrenia is like these genetic diseases, is quite different from saying there is a genetic predisposition to a developmental anomaly or to a viral infection. It is the difference between saying that the genetic factor is necessary for the etiology of a disease or saying that a genetic predisposition increases the chances of getting that disease, but that genes by themselves are not sufficient or necessary to cause it. Dr. Malgene seems to slide back and forth across this spectrum without making clear distinctions.

Finally, Dr. Malgene implies that just because genes are important in determining normal personality traits, they are also likely to be important in the etiology of schizophrenia. This is a specious argument because schizophrenia is a brain disease, not a collection of personality traits. Genes may or may not play an important role in causing schizophrenia, but this has nothing to do with their role in determining normal personality traits.

I will turn my attention next to Dr. Daverus's presentation. And much of what I just said in criticism of Dr. Malgene applies equally well to Dr. Daverus. She lays out for us a variety of models in which viruses might cause a chronic infection of the central nervous system and the symptoms of schizophrenia. However, it is not a question of whether viruses *can* do such things, but rather whether viruses *do* do such things. And if they do, how often? Dr. Daverus mentions the data on birth seasonality in schizophrenia, but as she is aware, the excess winter–spring birth seasonality associated with schizophrenia accounts for no more than 10% of all individuals with schizophrenia.

I would like to add that even if the pestiviruses or other viruses are identified in the serum or cerebrospinal fluid of schizophrenics, that does not necessarily mean that the viruses are associated with the disease process. They could be reactivated by an altered immune system in the disease and their presence would then be merely an epiphenomenon. So I would ask Dr. Daverus: How do you know whether the putative viruses are causal or merely casual?

DR. MALGENE: I certainly agree with Dr. D'Velupmoni's remarks and would like to raise a few additional questions for Dr. Daverus. If viruses are truly implicated in many cases of this disease, wouldn't you expect to see more explicit neuropathology on MRI scans and in neuropathological research? For example, shouldn't there be prominent gliosis of the hippocampus–amygdala and not merely a nonspecific reduction in size?

I am also puzzled by how Dr. Daverus can account for the evidence of widespread cerebral dysfunction in the twins. Both the neurological and the neuropsychological findings suggest a broad, scattered type of dysfunction rather than a focal type. Many neuroviruses primarily attack one specific area (e.g., rabies) or one specific cell type (e.g., polio), but in schizophrenia there is no evidence of such localization.

Finally, I would offer a brief comment on those cases of schizophrenia in this study that began immediately following an infection. If you take any illness, you can find such preceding infections because they are so ubiquitous. Although such individual cases are interesting, it is noteworthy that no single type of infection was found to occur in an unusual incidence in the twins prior to the onset of their schizophrenia.

DR. DAVERUS: I would like to offer a few comments on Dr. D'Velupmoni's theory of schizophrenia. It is a difficult theory to criticize because it has so many parts. It reminds me of the game we used to play at birthday parties when I was a child in which everybody won and therefore everybody got a prize. The developmental theory is like that—everybody will turn out to be right because almost everything can cause the putative brain lesion.

But let's think more clearly about this theory. It postulates the damage as taking place early in the course of brain development. And yet known causes of brain damage early in development, such as chromosomal abnormalities or metabolic diseases, usually cause mental retardation, not schizophrenia. And if the brain damage really takes place so early in development, wouldn't we expect developmental markers, such as minor physical anomalies and dermatoglyphic changes, to be much more prominent?

Another problem with the developmental theory is epidemiological. The areas of the world where there is the worst prenatal care and the highest occurrence of malnutrition of pregnant women, obstetrical complications, and postnatal infections are the developing nations. The developmental theory would predict that increased incidence of developmental insults should produce an increase of schizophrenia in such countries. Yet there is no evidence for this, and, in fact, what evidence exists points in the opposite direction: that schizophrenia has a *lower* incidence in developing nations.

DR. MALGENE: Along those same lines, I would like to focus on the nature of the insults. Many of the theoretical insults that can disrupt brain development and lead to late schizophrenia, such as decreased oxygen supply, are also thought to cause epilepsy and cerebral palsy. If, in fact, these insults are the original cause of schizophrenia, shouldn't epilepsy and cerebral palsy co-occur with schizophrenia more often than by chance? There is an example of one such case (cerebral palsy in one twin, schizoaffective disorder in the other) among the twins in this study, but I would expect a much higher incidence.

Where Do We Go from Here? To close the fictional discussion, the three experts were asked to state briefly what they believed to be the most important next steps to be taken for a better understanding of the cause of schizophrenia.

DR. MALGENE: Well, I think that the most important steps have already been taken by the support of multicenter molecular genetics studies in Europe and in the United States. In Europe, 18 centers, supported by the European Science Foundation, have been coordinating efforts for over 3 years to look for loci associated with schizophrenia and bipolar disorder by using 150 genetic markers spread across all chromosomes. A similar multicenter study is under way in the United States, supported by the National Institute of Mental Health. Such linkage studies assume that one or more major genes are important etiological factors.

Alternatively, there are those of us who favor a theory of polygenic inheritance of schizophrenia without the involvement of a major gene. We are counting on association strategies, in which different alleles of a genetic marker (i.e., occurring alternatively) are studied in individuals with schizophrenia and in normal controls, for the answers. The problem with this strategy, however, is that we still have not identified genetic markers that are essential for these strategies. I would therefore strongly support continued research on dopamine and other neurotransmitters in hopes that one or more of them will be found to be a genetic marker. Linkage and association strategies are the psychiatric wave of the future, and the research leaders of the next decade will be molecular geneticists.

Dr. Daverus: Viruses as possible etiological agents for schizophrenia and bipolar disorder have been greatly underresearched. That is now starting to change, primarily with the fiscal support of the Theodore and Vada Stanley Foundation. The increasing realization that the HIV virus, which causes AIDS, also causes widespread pathology in the central nervous system has increased interest in this field. Studies that have linked exposure to influenza in the middle trimester of pregnancy to the development of schizophrenia in the offspring many years later have also helped bring neurovirology into psychiatry.

The future holds great promise. Answers are likely to come from studies of serum, lymphocytes, cerebrospinal fluid, and postmortem brain tissue from individuals with schizophrenia. Personally, I suspect that viruses are also involved in the etiology of most cases of bipolar disorder as well, although a genetic predisposition appears to be more prominent in bipolar disorder than it is in schizophrenia. Another important research area will be the study of mothers during pregnancy and of infants in their first months of life, for those may be the periods when the virus that causes schizophrenia is transmitted. Future psychiatric researchers, then, will be experts in both neurovirology and perinatology, and the future schizophrenia research team may be centered in the departments of infectious disease and/or pediatrics.

Dr. D'Velupmoni: I'm afraid that I cannot share the optimism of my colleagues that either molecular genetics or virology will give us the answers. Schizophrenia probably involves many different factors, any one of which can impair the development of the brain at crucial stages of growth and thereby lead to later dysfunction.

The answers to this disease, therefore, are going to come more slowly as we gain a better understanding of brain development. We need to support more basic research—neuroanatomical, neurochemical and embryological—on how normal brains develop and function. This should also include more research on animal models of normal and abnormal brain development. Only when we have gone through the tedious but necessary steps of understanding this normal development will we be able to understand what goes wrong in the developmental process to produce schizophrenia. The future leadership of psychiatric research, therefore, will be in the hands of the neuroanatomists and other basic brain researchers.

Onward

Someone had to have the last word. The nonfictional counterparts of the cast of characters above have worked collaboratively and productively on the twin study for the past 7 years and the work continues.

And so these men of Industan disputed loud and long,

Each in his own opinion exceeding stiff and strong,

Though each was partly in the right,

And all were in the wrong!

[Old Indian legend]

REFERENCES

Andreasen, N. C. (1989). *Brain imaging: Applications in psychiatry.* (Washington, DC: American Psychiatric Press.

Barnard, E. A. (1992). GABA receptor genes: Applications to neuropsychiatric disorders. In J. Mendlewicz & H. Hippius (Eds.), *Genetic research in psychiatry.* Berlin: Springer-Verlag.

Berg, K. (1990). Level genes and variability genes in the etiology of hyperlipidemia and atherosclerosis. In K. Berg, N. Retterstol, & S. Refsum (Eds.), *From phenotype to gene in common disorders.* Copenhagen: Munksgaard.

Bertelsen, A., & Gottesman, I. I. (1990). Offspring of twins with schizophrenia: In reply. *Archives of General Psychiatry, 47,* 977–978.

Brown, Z. A., Benedetti, J., Ashley, R., *et al.* (1991). Neonatal herpes simplex virus infection in relation to asymptomatic maternal infection at the time of labor. *New England Journal of Medicine, 324,* 1247–1252.

Burke, W., & Motulsky, A. G. (1992). Hypertension. In R. A. King, J. I. Rotter, & A. G. Motulsky (Eds.), *The genetic basis of common diseases.* London: Oxford University Press.

Cadoret, R. J. (1973). Toward a definition of the schizoid state: Evidence from studies of twins and their families. *British Journal of Psychiatry, 122,* 679–685.

Claridge, G. (1994). A single indicator of risk for schizophrenia: Probable fact or likely myth? *Schizophrenia Bulletin, 20,* 151–168.

Coon, H., Byerley, W., Holik, J., *et al.* (1993). Linkage analysis of schizophrenia with five dopamine receptor genes in nine pedigrees. *American Journal of Human Genetics, 52,* 327–334.

Coon, H., Jensen, S., Holik, J., *et al.* (1994). Genomic scan for genes predisposing to schizophrenia. *American Journal of Medical Genetics (Neuropsychiatric Genetics), 54,* 59–71.

Crow, T. J. (1990). Nature of the genetic contribution to psychotic illness—A continuum viewpoint. *Acta Psychiatrica Scandinavica, 81,* 401–408.

Crow, T. J. (1994). Prenatal exposure to influenza as a cause of schizophrenia. *British Journal of Psychiatry, 164,* 588–592.

Davison, K. (1992). Organic schizophrenia-like psychoses. *Neurological Psychiatry and Brain Research, 1,* 90–94.

Day, R. (1986). Social stress and schizophrenia: From the concept of recent life events to the notion of toxic environments. In G. D. Burrows & T. R. Norman (Eds.), *Handbook of studies on schizophrenia.* Amsterdam: Elsevier.

Devereux, R. B., & Brown, W. T. (1992). Structural heart disease. In R. A. King, J. I. Rotter, & A. G. Motulsky, (Eds.), *The genetic basis of common diseases.* London: Oxford University Press.

Ehrnst, A., Lindgren, S., Dictor, M., *et al.* (1991). HIV in pregnant women and their offspring: Evidence for late transmission. *Lancet, 338,* 203–207.

Essen-Moller, E., Larsson, H., Uddenberg, C. E., *et al.* (1956). Individual traits and morbidity in a Swedish rural population. *Acta Psychiatrica et Neurologica Scandinavica* (Suppl. 100).

Farmer, A. E., McGuffin, P., & Gottesman, I. I. (1987). Twin concordance for DSM-III schizophrenia: Scrutinizing the validity of the definition. *Archives of General Psychiatry, 44,* 634–641.

Fischer, M. (1971). Psychoses in the offspring of schizophrenic monozygotic twins and their normal co-twins. *British Journal of Psychiatry, 118,* 43–52.

Gershon, E. S., & Cloninger, C. R. (1994). *Genetic approaches to mental disorders.* Washington, DC: American Psychiatric Press.

Gottesman, I. I. (1987). The psychotic hinterlands or the fringes of lunacy. *British Medical Bulletin, 43,* 557–569.

Gottesman, I. I. (1991). *Schizophrenia genesis—The origins of madness.* San Francisco: Freeman.

Gottesman, I. I. (1994a). Complications to the complex inheritance of schizophrenia. *Clinical Genetics, 46,* 116–123.

Gottesman, I. I. (1994b). Schizophrenia epigenesis: Past, present, and future. *Acta Psychiatrica Scandinavica, 90*(Suppl. 384), 26–33.

Gottesman, I. I., & Bertelsen, A. (1989). Confirming unexpressed genotypes for schizophrenia. Risks in the offspring of Fischer's Danish identical and fraternal discordant twins. *Archives of General Psychiatry, 46,* 867–872.

Gottesman, I. I., & McGue, P. M. (1991). Mixed and mixed-up models for the transmission of schizophrenia. In W. Grove & D. Cicchetti (Eds.), *Thinking clearly about psychology: Personality and psychopathology* (Vol. 2). Minneapolis: University of Minnesota Press.

Gottesman, I. I., & Shields, J. (1967). A polygenic theory of schizophrenia. *Proceedings of the National Academy of Sciences USA, 58,* 199–205.

Gottesman, I. I., & Shields, J. (1972). *Schizophrenia and genetics: A twin study vantage point.* New York: Academic Press.

Heston, L. L. (1966). Psychiatric disorders in the foster home reared children of schizophrenic mothers. *British Journal of Psychiatry, 112,* 819–825.

Huntington's Disease Collaborative Research Group. (1993). A novel gene containing a trinucleotide repeat that is expanded and unstable on the Huntington's disease chromosome. *Cell, 72,* 971–983.

Iacono, W. G., & Clementz, B. A. (1993). A strategy for elucidating genetic influences on complex psychopathological syndromes (with special reference to ocular motor functioning and schizophrenia). *Progress in Experimental Personality and Psychopathology Research, 16,* 11–65.

Jablensky, A. (1993). The epidemiology of schizophrenia. *Current Opinion in Psychiatry, 6,* 43–52.

Kendler, K. S., & Diehl, S. R. (1993). The genetics of schizophrenia: A current, genetic-epidemiologic perspective. *Schizophrenic Bulletin, 19,* 261–285.

Kendler, K. S., Gruenberg, A. M., & Kinney, D. K. (1994). Independent diagnoses of adoptees and relatives, using DSM-III criteria in the provincial and national samples of the Danish Adoption Study of Schizophrenia. *Archives of General Psychiatry, 51,* 456–468.

Kendler, K. S., McGuire, M., Gruenberg, A. M., *et al.* (1993). The Roscommon family study: I. Methods, diagnosis of probands and risk of schizophrenia in relatives. *Archives of General Psychiatry, 50,* 527–540.

Kety, S. S., Wender, P. H., Jacobsen, B., *et al.* (1994). Mental illness in the biological and adoptive relatives of schizophrenic adoptees: Replication of the Copenhagen study in the rest of Denmark. *Archives of General Psychiatry, 51,* 442–455.

King, R. A., Rotter, J. I., & Motulsky, A. G. (Eds.). (1992). *The genetic basis of common diseases.* London: Oxford University Press.

Kringlen, E., & Cramer, G. (1989). Offspring of monozygotic twins discordant for schizophrenia. *Archives of General Psychiatry, 46,* 873–877.

Lenzenweger, M. F. (1993). Explorations in schizotypy and the psychometric high-risk para-digm. *Progress in Experimental Personality and Psychopathology Research, 16,* 66–116.

Lipska, B. K., Jaskiw, G. E., & Weinberger, D. R. (1993). Postpubertal emergence of hyper-responsiveness to stress and to amphetamine after neonatal excitotoxic hippocampal damage: A potential animal model of schizophrenia. *Neuropsychopharmacology, 9,* 67–75.

McGue, M. (1992). When assessing twin concordance, use the probandwise not the pairwise rate. *Schizophrenia Bulletin, 18,* 171–176.

McGuffin, P., Katz, R., Rutherford, J., et al. (1993). Twin studies as vital indicators of pheno-types in molecular genetic research. In T. J. Bouchard & P. Propping (Eds.), *Twins as a tool of behavioral genetics.* New York: Wiley.

McGuffin, P., Owen, M. J., O'Donovan, M. C., et al., (1994). *Seminars in psychiatric genetics.* London: Gaskell Press.

Maier, W., Lichtermann, D., Hallmayer, J., et al. (1993). Continuity and discontinuity of affective disorders and schizophrenia: Results of a controlled family study. *Archives of General Psychiatry, 50,* 871–883.

Mednick, S. (Ed.). (1995). *Neural development in schizophrenia: Theory and research.* New York: Plenum Press.

Mendlewicz, J., & Hippius, H. (Eds.). (1992). *Genetic research in psychiatry.* Berlin: Springer-Verlag.

Moldin, S. O., & Gottesman, I. I. (1995). Population genetics in psychiatry. In H. I. Kaplan & B. J. Sadock (Eds.), *Comprehensive textbook of psychiatry* (6th ed.). Baltimore: Williams & Wilkins, pp. 144–155.

Moldin, S. O., Gottesman, I. I., Erlenmeyer-Kimling, L., et al. (1990). Psychometric deviance in offspring at risk for schizophrenia: I. Initial delineation of a distinct subgroup. *Psychiatry Research, 32,* 297–310.

Motulsky, A. G., & Brunzell, J. D. (1992). The genetics of coronary atherosclerosis. In R. A. King, J. I. Rotter, & A. G. Motulsky (Eds.), *The genetic basis of common diseases.* London: Oxford University Press.

Nowakowski, R. S. (1987). Basic concepts of CNS development. *Child Development, 58,* 568–595.

Odegaard, O. (1952). La Genetique Dans la Psychiatrie. *Proceedings of the First World Congress in Psychiatry, VI,* 84–90.

Odegaard, O. (1972). The multifactorial theory of inheritance in predisposition to schizophre-nia. In A. R. Kaplan (Ed.), *Genetic factors in schizophrenia.* Springfield, IL: CC Thomas.

Oldstone, M. B. A., Sinha, Y. N., Blount, P., et al. (1982). Virus-induced alterations in homeostasis: Alterations in differentiated functions of infected cells in vivo. *Science, 218,* 1125–1127.

Onstad, S., Skre, I., Torgersen, S., et al. (1991). Twin concordance for DSM-III-R schizophrenia. *Acta Psychiatrica Scandinavica, 83,* 395–401.

Owen, M. J. (1992). Will schizophrenia become a graveyard for molecular geneticists? *Psycho-logical Medicine, 22,* 289–293.

Peters, C. J., Reeves, W. C., & Purcell, R. H. (1977). Disparate response of monozygotic twins to hepatitis B virus infection. *Journal of Pediatrics, 91,* 265–266.

Prescott, C. A., & Gottesman, I. I. (1993). Genetically mediated vulnerability to schizophrenia. *Psychiatric Clinics of North America, 16,* 245–267.

Roos, R. P. (1985). Genetically controlled resistance to viral infections of the central nervous system. *Progress in Medical Genetics, 6,* 242–276.

Saugstad, L., & Odegaard, O. (1986). Huntington's chorea in Norway. *Psychological Medicine, 16,* 39–48.

Sierra-Honigmann, A. M., Carbone, K. M., & Yolken, R. H. (1995). Polymerase chain reaction (PCR) search for the viral nucleic acid sequences in schizophrenia. *British Journal of Psychiatry, 166,* 55–60.

Sing, C. F., & Moll, P. P. (1990). Strategies for unravelling the genetic basis of coronary artery disease. In K. Berg, N. Retterstol, & S. Refsum (Eds.), *From phenotype to gene in common disorders.* Copenhagen: Munksgaard.

Sobell, J. L., Heston, L. L., & Sommer, S. S. (1993). Novel association approach for determining the genetic predisposition to schizophrenia: Case–control resource and resting of a candidate gene. *American Journal of Medical Genetics (Neuropsychiatric Genetics), 48,* 28–35.

Stromgren, E. (1987). Changes in the incidence of schizophrenia. *British Journal of Psychiatry, 150,* 1–7.

Stromgren, E. (1994). The unitary psychosis (Einheitspsychose) concept: Past and present. *Neurology, Psychiatry, & Brain Research, 2,* 201–205.

Thaler, M. M., Park, C. K., Landers, D. V., et al. (1991). Vertical transmission of hepatitis C virus. *Lancet, 338,* 17–18.

Tienari, P. J., Wikstrom, J., Sajantila, A., et al. (1992). Genetic susceptibility to multiple sclerosis linked to myelin basic protein gene. *Lancet, 340,* 987–991.

Tienari, P., Wynne, L., Moring, J., et al. (1994). The Finnish Adoptive Family Study of Schizophrenia: A longitudinal study exploring joint effects of genetics and environment. *Acta Psychiatrica Scandinavica (Suppl.).*

Torrey, E. F. (1989). Schizophrenia: Fixed incidence or fixed thinking? *Psychological Medicine, 19,* 285–287.

Torrey, E. F. (1991). A viral-anatomical explanation of schizophrenia. *Schizophrenia Bulletin, 17*(1), 15–18.

Torrey, E. F. (1992). Are we overestimating the genetic contribution to schizophrenia? *Schizophrenia Bulletin, 18,* 159–170.

Torrey, E. F. (1995). *Surviving schizophrenia: A manual for families, consumers, and providers* (3rd ed.). New York: Harper & Row.

Torrey, E. F., Bowler, A. E., Taylor, E. H., & Gottesman, I. I. (1994). *Schizophrenia and manic-depressive disorder: The biological roots of mental illness as revealed by the landmark study of identical twins.* New York: Basic Books.

Tsujita, T., Okazaki, Y., Fujimara, K., et al. (1992). *Twin concordance rate of DSM-III schizophrenia in a new Japanese sample.* Unpublished manuscript.

Walker, E. (1994). Developmentally moderated expressions of the neuropathology underlying schizophrenia. *Schizophrenia Bulletin, 20,* 453–480.

Warner, R. (1994). *Recovery from schizophrenia—Psychiatry and political economy.* New York: Routledge.

Weinberger, D. R. (1987). Implications of normal brain development for the pathogenesis of schizophrenia. *Archives of General Psychiatry, 44,* 660–669.

Whitaker, J. N., Sever, J. L., & Engel, W. K. (1972). Subacute sclerosing panencephalitis in only one of identical twins. *New England Journal of Medicine, 287,* 864–866.

CHAPTER 5

The Inheritance
of Mood Disorders

MING T. TSUANG and STEPHEN V. FARAONE

In this chapter we will show that although much is known about the inheritance of mood disorders, we still have much to learn. Available studies weave a complex pattern of results that inform clinicians, educate students, and stimulate researchers. A complete review of relevant work is beyond the scope of a single chapter; those who wish to learn more should consult comprehensive reviews (Faraone, Kremen, & Tsuang, 1990; Tsuang and Faraone, 1990) along with the original studies. Our goal for this chapter is to provide an overview that orients readers to basic findings and future directions. However, before doing so, we briefly review the spectrum of conditions called *mood disorders* to create a nosological foundation for the studies to be reviewed.

MING T. TSUANG • Harvard Institute of Psychiatric Epidemiology and Genetics; Harvard Medical School Department of Psychiatry at the Massachusetts Mental Health Center and Brockton/West Roxbury VA Medical Center; and Department of Epidemiology, Harvard School of Public Health, Boston, Massachusetts 02115.   STEPHEN V. FARAONE • Harvard Institute of Psychiatric Epidemiology and Genetics; Harvard Medical School Department of Psychiatry at the Massachusetts Mental Health Center and Brockton/West Roxbury VA Medical Center; and Pediatric Psychopharmacology Unit, Psychiatry Service, Massachusetts General Hospital, Boston, Massachusetts 02114.
Genetics and Mental Illness: Evolving Issues for Research and Society, edited by Laura Lee Hall. Plenum Press, New York, 1996.

THE DIAGNOSIS OF MOOD DISORDERS

Disorders of mood range from an extreme state of elation known as mania, to a severe state of dysphoria known as depression. Because these disorders are clinically heterogeneous, there have been several attempts to create meaningful subgroups. Our goal in reviewing some of these subgroupings is to illustrate how nosologists have conceptualized the mood disorders—not to present one diagnostic approach as superior to others. As we discuss in detail elsewhere (Tsuang, Faraone, & Lyons, 1993), the adequacy of a diagnostic approach cannot be divorced from its proposed use. Thus, a diagnostic system useful for genetic studies may not be useful in a clinical setting (and vice versa).

Unipolar Depression versus Bipolar Mood Disorders

Perhaps the most obvious means of subclassifying the mood disorders is according to the type of mood disturbance. Initially, psychiatric nosology recognized a broad class of illness known as *manic-depressive psychosis.* However, much research suggested that it would be useful to separate the "manic" and "depressive" components when classifying mood-disordered patients.

In this approach, unipolar depressive disorder is diagnosed when the patient experiences only depressive episodes; bipolar disorder is warranted when the patient experiences both manic and depressive episodes. (Patients who have experienced only manic episodes are rare and are usually classified as having bipolar disorder because research indicates that most will eventually have a depressive episode.)

The bipolar group is further subdivided into three categories based on the severity of the manic episode: bipolar I patients have had at least one episode of mania, bipolar II (or hypomanic) patients have had manic symptoms but not a full manic episode, and bipolar III patients have had only depressive episodes yet have at least one biological relative with a history of mania.

To assess the validity of the unipolar–bipolar distinction, researchers have examined demographic variables, psychopathology, clinical course, response to medication, and biochemical variables (Tsuang & Faraone, 1990). Unipolar patients usually have later age at onset than bipolar patients. Also, whereas bipolar disorder is equally common among males and females, unipolar disorder is approximately twice as prevalent among females than males. Furthermore, unipolar depression is associated with higher levels of psychomotor agitation (excessive motor activity associated with a feeling of inner tension). In contrast, psychomotor retardation is observed among bipolar depressives. Compared with bipolar patients, unipolar patients are more likely to complain of somatic problems and to express anger. Also, bipolar depressed patients usually experience hypersomnia whereas unipolar depressives complain of insomnia.

Studies of pharmacologic response have also examined the unipolar–bipolar distinction. Lithium carbonate is well known for its therapeutic and prophylactic effects in the treatment of mania but is also an effective treatment for depression. Furthermore, antidepressant medication has been shown to be effective in preventing depressive episodes for both bipolar and unipolar patients. Similarly, although some biochemical differences between unipolar and bipolar patients have been demonstrated, consistent differences that reliably discriminate the two disorders have not been reported.

Endogenous versus Reactive Depression

"Endogenous" depressive episodes are those that appear unrelated to environmental events whereas "reactive" depressions display a chronic course of less severe, stress-related episodes. The most consistent difference between endogenous and reactive depressives is in their clinical phenomenology. Endogenous depression is associated with early morning waking, psychomotor retardation, severely depressed mood, feelings of guilt, remorse, and worthlessness, difficulty concentrating, loss of interest, and weight change. In contrast, reactive depressions show late night insomnia, feelings of self-pity, and anxiety. Response to treatment has also been used to compare endogenous and reactive depressions. The most consistent finding is that, in comparison to nonendogenous depressives, endogenous depressives have a better response to tricyclic antidepressant medication and a worse response to psychotherapy. Endogenous depressives are more likely to receive electroconvulsive therapy and are more likely to benefit from such therapy.

Primary versus Secondary Mood Disorders

Mood disorders are known to occur in the context of many other psychiatric conditions. For example, a post-psychotic depression commonly affects schizophrenic patients (Tsuang & Faraone, 1994). Patients with alcoholism, somatoform disorders, and anxiety disorders have also been observed to manifest depressive syndromes. Depressive episodes preceded by another psychiatric condition have been called *secondary depressions,* a term that implies that they may have been caused by the other condition. Although secondary depressives may not differ from primary depressives in their clinical phenomenology, some studies suggest that the course and outcome of secondary cases would be determined by the nature of the concomitant disorder.

The primary–secondary distinction, although usually applied to depression, is also applicable to the classification of mania. This is especially true when the group of secondary mood disorders is extended to include depression and mania in the context of physical disease. Mania has been associated with viral infection, surgical procedures, cerebral tumors, multiple sclerosis, and head injuries. Depression may also be related to nonpsychiatric disease. Whitlock (1982) estimated that, among patients with severe depression, 20–30% can be attributed to physical conditions such as presenile dementia, infections, cerebral tumors, epilepsy, cancer, and immunologic diseases.

The primary–secondary distinction is crucial for genetic studies. Clearly, mood disorders secondary to physical disease may be cases that mimic a genetic disorder. These "phenocopies" may distort the results of genetic epidemiologic research. In contrast, the status of mood disorders secondary to other psychiatric disorders is less clear because the co-occurrence of psychiatric disorders is fairly common. From an epidemiologic study of over 11,000 people, Boyd *et al.* (1984) concluded that the presence of any psychiatric disorder increased the odds of having other disorders. For example, a person with major depression had about 19 times the odds of having panic disorder compared with nondepressed individuals. Other disorders found to co-occur with major depression were agoraphobia, simple phobia, obsessive-compulsive disorder, schizophrenia, somatization disorder, antisocial personality, and substance abuse or dependence. The National Comorbidity Survey recently reported high levels of comorbidity in another large population sample: 27% of individuals met criteria for two or more psychiatric disorders (Kessler *et al.,* 1994). Among 394 subjects who reported a current episode of major depression, 56% had a comorbid psychiatric disorder (Blazer, Kessler, McGonagle, & Swartz, 1994). Thus, psychiatric comorbidity may be the rule, rather than the exception for major depressive disorder.

Schizoaffective Disorder

Traditionally, nosologic thinking in psychiatry has separated mood disorders from schizophrenia. The latter is a heterogeneous condition characterized by hallucinations, delusions, disordered thinking, and poor social adjustment (Tsuang & Faraone, 1994). Nevertheless, some psychotic patients do not fit neatly into either category. We call these patients "schizoaffective" because they experience the perceptual and cognitive abnormalities of schizophrenia along with disorders of mood and associated characteristics of mood disorders (Marneros & Tsuang, 1986).

Taken as a whole, relevant research strongly supports the claim that schizoaffective disorder is related to both schizophrenia and mood disorders (Tsuang & Faraone, 1990). Available data support four empirical generalizations: (1) schizoaffective symptomatology is a mix of mood and schizophrenic disorder symptoms; (2) the schizoaffective pattern of course does not differ greatly from those of schizophrenic and mood disorders; (3) on average, the outcome of schizoaffective disorder is intermediate in severity relative to the other psychoses; and (4) the treatment regime for schizoaffective disorder consists of treatments used for schizophrenic and mood disorders.

Current Nomenclature

Three diagnostic systems are frequently used in psychiatric research: the Washington University (WU) Criteria (Feighner *et al.*, 1972); the Research Diagnostic Criteria (RDC) (Spitzer, Endicott, & Robins, 1978), and the fourth edition of the *Diagnostic and Statistical Manual* (DSM-IV) (American Psychiatric Association, 1994), the official diagnostic manual of the American Psychiatric Association. The WU system includes three mood disorder diagnoses: primary mania, primary depression, and secondary depression. The criteria for mania require a period of euphoria or irritability in the context of a psychiatric disorder lasting at least 2 weeks. In addition, the patient must exhibit at least three of six manic symptoms and may be excluded from the diagnosis by evidence of preexisting psychiatric conditions or a prominence of schizophrenic-like psychotic symptoms. The criteria for primary depression require an episode of dysphoric mood in the context of a psychiatric disorder lasting at least 1 month. Five of eight depressive symptoms must be present and, in addition to the manic exclusion criteria, the diagnosis is excluded if the depressive syndrome is preceded by a serious medical illness. The WU diagnosis of secondary depression selects patients with preexisting nonmood psychiatric disorder or serious medical illness who meet the nonexclusionary criteria for primary depression.

The RDC criteria cover a wider spectrum of mood disorders than the WU criteria. These are manic disorder, major depressive disorder, bipolar

I disorder, bipolar II disorder, hypomanic disorder, minor depressive disorder, intermittent depressive disorder, and cyclothymic personality. RDC criteria for mania are very similar to WU criteria with four differences. RDC requires only 1 week (instead of 2 weeks) of symptoms and includes poor judgment as a manic symptom. Also, the RDC requires that the manic disturbance be "severe" and does not exclude patients with preexisting psychiatric disorders other than schizophrenia.

The RDC criteria for major depressive disorder also differ from WU primary depression. RDC requires only 2 weeks (instead of 1 month) of symptoms and includes a severity of disturbance requirement. Unlike the WU system, RDC does not exclude patients with preexisting psychiatric disturbances other than schizophrenia. Moreover, criteria for ten subtypes of major depressive disorder are provided by RDC. Additional RDC mood disorder diagnoses deal with combinations of manic and depressive symptoms, schizoaffective disorders, and syndromes of lesser severity. Bipolar I disorder indicates a history of manic disorder and major depressive disorder, minor depressive disorder, or intermittent depressive disorder. Bipolar II disorder requires a history positive for both hypomanic disorder and major, minor, or intermittent depressive disorder [hypomanic disorder is essentially a mild version of manic disorder, only two manic symptoms are required (three if mood is only irritable), and the duration of the mood disturbance is only 2 days].

RDC minor depressive disorder is similar to major depressive disorder, but requires the presence of only two depressive symptoms from a larger symptom list including relatively mild experiences such as pessimistic attitude and self-pity. Minor depression does not require impairment in functioning or referral for psychiatric services. Intermittent depressive disorder is diagnosed when there are no clear-cut episodes of a sustained depressive mood but the patient has been bothered periodically by depressed mood for at least 2 years. The category of cyclothymic personality is reserved for patients who experience recurrent periods of depression lasting at least several days alternating with periods of notably good mood characterized by at least two of the symptoms seen in hypomanic disorder. The periods of mood change must have been present since the early 20s and must be too numerous to count (i.e., the patient is rarely in a normal mood).

The DSM-IV criteria for mania and depression are similar to the RDC criteria. Patients experiencing a DSM-IV manic episode are diagnosed bipolar disorder, mixed if their current episode involves the full symptomatic picture of both mania and depression. They are diagnosed bipolar I disorder, manic if their current or most recent episode was a manic episode. Patients meeting criteria for a DSM-IV depressive episode are classified as bipolar I disorder, depressed if they have had one or more manic episodes in the past. Otherwise they are classified as major depression, single episode, or major depression, recurrent, depending on the number of depressive episodes in their history. If a patient with a major depressive history also has a history including some manic features (hypomanic) but not a full manic episode, he or she is classified as bipolar II.

In DSM-IV, schizoaffective disorder is diagnosed if the patient experiences a full depressive or manic syndrome concurrently with the psychotic symptoms characteristic of schizophrenia. The diagnosis of schizophrenia must first be ruled out and the patient must have had an episode including delusions or hallucinations for at least 2 weeks without prominent mood symptoms. The DSM-IV diagnosis of schizoaffective disorder is explicitly longitudinal. That is, one must observe the relative prominence of psychotic and mood symptoms over time before a diagnosis can be definitely established.

DSM-IV also includes diagnostic categories for affective disorders that are less severe than bipolar disorder or major depression. Individuals who meet neither bipolar nor major depressive diagnoses will be classified as having cyclothymic disorder if they have at least a 2-year history of numerous periods during which some of the characteristic symptoms of depression and mania were evident. The symptomatic periods may be separated by periods of normal mood lasting as long as 2 months. Dysthymic disorder is diagnosed in an individual with at least a 2-year history of symptoms characteristic of the depressive syndrome who does not meet the criteria for a major depressive episode. Periods of normal mood may last a few days to a few weeks but no more than 2 months at a time for this diagnosis. Depressive disorder not otherwise specified will be diagnosed in an individual who exhibits depressive symptoms without meeting the criteria for any specific mood disorder.

GENETIC STUDIES OF MOOD DISORDERS

For the genetic epidemiologist, the distribution of illness within families provides clues about the effects and interactions of genes and environment. Genetic epidemiologic studies thus use different family structures to answer specific questions. Studies of nuclear and extended families indicate if a disorder is familial, i.e., that it "runs in families." However, such studies cannot disentangle the relative contributions of genetic and environmental factors. To do so we must consult twin and adoption studies. After establishing that genetic factors play a role, the next task is to determine the mode of transmission and, eventually, the genetic and environmental mechanisms of the disease. We provide a detailed discussion of these methodologies elsewhere (Faraone & Santangelo, 1992; Faraone & Tsuang, 1994).

Family Studies of Mood Disorders

If genes cause mood disorders, then the relatives of mood-disorderd patients should have a greater risk for the illness than the relatives of nonpatients. Genetic epidemiologists use the term *proband* to designate patients and nonpatients who are initially selected for a family study. Following biological laws of inheritance, the risk to relatives of probands is directly related to the amount of genes they share with the proband. Relatives who share 50% of their genes with the proband (i.e., parents, children, and siblings) are known as first-degree relatives. Relatives who share only 25% of the genes with the proband (grandparents, uncles, aunts, nephews, and nieces) are second-degree relatives.

If a mood disorder is genetically transmitted, first-degree relatives of probands should have higher rates of mood disorders than second-degree relatives (because the former share a higher percentage of genes than the latter). In short, the hypothesis that genes predispose to illness predicts that the relatives of mood-disordered probands are at a greater risk for the disorder than are the relatives of control probands and that the risk to relatives of ill probands decreases based on the percentage of genes they have in common. That is, individuals who are more distantly related to an ill proband will be at lower risk for the disorder than those who are closely related to an ill proband.

Although genetic hypotheses predict that disorders will be familial, familiality can have other causes. For example, family members share a common culture and a common environment and the similarity of these factors tends to increase as the degree of the relationship decreases. Thus, familial environmental factors may confound genetic relationships. For example, if cigarette smoking is a habit that children learn from parents, then one might observe that smoking-related disorders run in families. In this case, familial transmission results primarily from relatives sharing a common environmental pathogen. Possible sources of cultural and environmental transmission include bacteria, viruses, learned responses to stress, cultural differences in emotional expression, and others.

Before examining family studies of mood disorders, it is useful to examine population-based epidemiologic data (Tsuang & Faraone, 1990). Such studies are useful in this regard because they provide a context in which family study data can be interpreted. Early epidemiologic studies of "manic-depressive psychosis," performed from 1938 to 1952, found the risk for the illness in the general population to range from 0.4 to 1.7%. The mean risk was 0.7%. Relatively recent epidemiologic studies separate cases according to the unipolar–bipolar distinction. In these studies lifetime rates of bipolar disorder ranged from 0.1 to 1.6%. Thus, the population risks for bipolar disorder are similar to the risks reported for manic-depressive psychosis from earlier studies. In contrast, rates of unipolar disorder in the general population were much higher, ranging from 3.4 to 18.0%. All of these studies that examined unipolar and bipolar disorders find a greater prevalence of unipolar disorder.

Early family studies of mood disorders were conducted from 1929 to 1954. They did not make the distinction between unipolar and bipolar disorders and only report the risk for manic-depression among relatives of manic-depressive probands (Tsuang & Faraone, 1990). The risk to parents ranged from 3.2 to 23.4% with a mean of 14.6%. The risk to siblings ranged from 2.7 to 23.0% with a mean of 10.9%. Each of the studies found relatives of mood-disordered probands to be at greater risk for manic-depressive psychosis than the 0.7% general population risk reported by the early epidemiologic studies.

Family studies performed during the past three decades benefited from an increased rigor of scientific methods and writing. Some of these studies address issues of potential diagnostic bias by making the interviewer "blind" to the diagnoses of the interviewees' relatives. Also, many of these later studies presented results separately for unipolar and bipolar subtypes; thus, they allowed the examination of the familial association of these two disorders.

The double-blind, controlled study of Gershon et al. (1982) examined 166 first-degree relatives of unipolar probands. Among these relatives, they found a 1.5% risk for bipolar disorder; this was greater than the 0.0% risk for controls but less than 4.5% risk for relatives of bipolar probands. The 16.6% risk of unipolar disorder to relatives of unipolar probands was not much greater than the 14.0% risk of unipolar disorder to relatives of bipolar probands but was nearly three times the risk observed in the control group. These results are similar to those of controlled studies of Tsuang, Winokur, and Crowe (1980) and Gershon et al. (1975); each of these studies found strong evidence for a familial component to unipolar disorder and weaker evidence of bipolar disorder to be elevated in unipolar families.

Weissman, Gershon, et al. (1984) studied the psychiatric disorders in 2003 first-degree relatives of 335 unipolar probands. Probands were diagnosed with structured personal interviews based on the research diagnostic criteria. Relatives were interviewed using the same diagnostic instrument based on the research diagnostic criteria along with family history evaluations from multiple informants. Approximately 75% of the evaluations of relatives were blind to proband diagnostic status. The researchers assessed a community sample of 82 normal controls with similar diagnostic methodologies. The 8.1% risk of bipolar disorder among relatives of unipolar probands was four times the risk observed in the community. The 18.4% risk of unipolar disorder was three times the risk reported in the community. Thus, consistent with other double-blind, controlled studies, there is evidence for a familial component to unipolar disorder, and some suggestion of a familial coaggregation of unipolar and bipolar disorders.

The study of Endicott *et al.* (1985) included 121 recurrent unipolar probands and their 424 first-degree relatives. The 0.7% risk of bipolar disorder among the relatives is not much greater than the population expectation and is less than the 2.3% reported for relatives of bipolar probands. The risk of unipolar disorder to relatives of unipolar probands (11.1%) was not much greater than the 8.3% risk to relatives of bipolar probands. The results from the NIMH Collaborative Study of Depression (Andreasen *et al.,* 1987) found a 0.6% risk of bipolar disorder and a 28.4% risk for unipolar disorder among relatives of unipolar probands. Although the unipolar diagnosis did not require recurrent episodes, the relatives' risk of bipolar disorder does not suggest a familial link between the two disorders. In contrast, the 28.4% risk of unipolar disorder provides strong evidence for familial transmission.

Sadovnick *et al.* (1994) used the family history method to diagnose 2913 family members of unipolar depressed patients and 781 relatives of bipolar patients. Among relatives of unipolar patients, 2.9% had a single depression, 2.6% had recurrent depression, and 0.7% had bipolar disorder. For relatives of bipolar patients the respective rates were 3.2, 2.2, and 4.1%. The relatively low rates in this study reflect the use of the family history method instead of direct interviews. Nevertheless, they are consistent with other work in finding bipolar disorder primarily among the relatives of bipolar, not unipolar, probands. In contrast, unipolar disorder was found in both types of families.

In summary, family studies of mood disorders consistently find that both unipolar and bipolar disorders "run in families." There is some indication of a genetic overlap between bipolar disorder and some cases of unipolar disorder, but further work is needed to clarify the nature and extent of this relationship.

Twin Studies of Mood Disorders

After the family study method has been used to establish that a disorder is familial, the next question is: "What are the relative contributions of genetic and environmental factors to disease etiology?" To answer this question it is necessary to go beyond family studies to twin and adoption studies.

Twinning provides a valuable opportunity to look at the factors involved in human genetics. Monozygotic (MZ) twins have 100% of their genes in common and dizygotic (DZ) twins, only 50%. Although the two types of twins are significantly different in terms of their genetic makeup, both MZ and DZ twins share a relatively common environment. The genetic similarity between DZ twins is the same as for any pair of siblings, but MZ twins are genetic copies of one another. Since DZ twins are not genetic copies of each other, differences within a DZ twin pair can be the result of either environmental or genetic factors. In contrast, environmental influences must be responsible for differences between MZ pairs. Thus, twins can be used to disentangle the relative contributions of genetic and environmental factors in the etiology of psychiatric disorders.

"Concordance" rates are often used to summarize twin studies of psychiatric disorders. A twin pair is concordant for illness if both twins are ill; if one is ill and the other well, the pair is discordant. If genetic factors are important and the effects of a common environment are the same for both types of twins, we expect a higher concordance rate for a disorder in MZ twins than in DZ twins.

In addition to concordance rates, we can estimate the heritability of a disorder from twin data. Heritability is a measure of the degree to which genetic factors influence the phenotypic variability of a disorder. Phenotypic variability (V_p) comprises two sources of variance: genetic variability (V_g) and environmental variability (V_e). Partitioning the phenotypic variability in this way assumes that genetic and environmental factors are statistically independent (i.e., $V_p = V_g + V_e$). Heritability in the broad sense (h^2) is the ratio of genetic and phenotypic variances (i.e., $h^2 = V_g/V_p$). Thus, a heritability of zero indicates that there is no genetic variability in the sample under consideration. That does not mean, however, that the etiology of the phenotype can be explained solely by environmental influence. Similarly, a heritability of one indicates that environmental factors are not relevant to disease etiology or that such factors have no variability in the sample under consideration.

A Danish twin study (Bertelsen, Harvald, & Hauge, 1977) identified twins through the Danish Psychiatric Twin Register. The investigators found a probandwise concordance rate for bipolar disorder of 0.67 in MZ twins, which was more than three times greater than DZ twins with a rate of 0.20. From these data, they calculated the heritability of mood disorder to be 0.59.

Tsuang and Faraone (1990) reviewed six twin studies of "manic-depressive disorder" that did not distinguish between unipolar and bipolar subforms. Overall, these studies attributed 60% of the variance in mood disorders to genetic factors; 30 to 40% of the variance was assigned to common environmental factors. Unique environmental effects accounted for less than 10% of the variance.

Since that review, additional twin studies have been performed. McGuffin, Katz, and Rutherford (1991) studied twins who had been systematically ascertained via 84 MZ and 130 DZ probands. For a lifetime history of "hospital-treated depression," concordance rates were 68% for MZ twins and 43% for DZ twins. A simple additive model suggested that 43% of the phenotypic variance could be attributed to genetic factors whereas 46% was assigned to common environment. For the DSM-III diagnosis of any lifetime major affective disorder, the MZ and DZ concordances were 53 and 28%, respectively. Model fitting assigned 51% of the variance of genetic factors and 31% to common environment.

Kendler, Neale, Kessler, Heath, and Eaves (1992) used a population-based study of 1033 twin pairs to examine the impact of nine different definitions of lifetime history of depression on the fit of genetic models. For all definitions, the best-fitting model assigned significant variance to additive genetic factors (21 to 45%) and individual-specific environmental factors (55 to 75%). In contrast, the effects of dominant genes and shared environment were not significant for any definition of depression. Similar results held for analyses of the 1-year prevalence of depression in this sample (Kendler, Neale, Kessler, Heath, & Eaves, 1993) and for analyses of varying definitions in a Swedish twin sample (Kendler, Pedersen, Johnson, Neale, & Mathe, 1993). Thus, this work suggests that genes account for all of the family resemblance observed in depression but also asserts that environmental factors play a substantial role in etiology.

In further discussions of their twin sample, Kendler, Kessler, *et al.* (1993) postulated there to be four key sources for the etiology of major depression in women: genetic factors, traumatic experiences, temperament, and interpersonal relations. Among these factors, stressful life events was the strongest predictor of depression. As regards genetic effects, approximately 60% of the effect was direct (i.e., not mediated by temperament or other factors). If confirmed by other studies, this work suggests that major depression is a multifactorial condition whose genetic causes may be overshadowed by environmental circumstances.

Overall, twin studies are consistent with family studies in suggesting that genetic factors play a substantial role in the mood disorders. However, the finding of MZ concordance rates lower than 100% documents the importance of environmental factors. These factors include sources of experimental error (e.g., psychiatric diagnostic, and zygosity misclassification).

Twin studies are less consistent in their attribution of environmental sources of variance to unique versus common environmental factors.

Adoption Studies of Mood Disorders

Like twin studies, adoption studies can disentangle genetic and environmental contributions to the familial transmission of a disorder. The adoption study capitalizes on two types of relationships: adoptive and biological. In doing so, it seeks to show whether genetic or adoptive (i.e., environmental) relationships account for the transmission of disorders. Clearly, children adopted at an early age have a primarily genetic relationship with their biological parents and an environmental relationship with their adoptive parents.

An adoption study from Belgium (Mendlewicz & Rainer, 1977) found the prevalence of psychiatric illness to be greater among the biological than the adoptive parents of bipolar adoptees. Compared with a control group, the biological parents of bipolar nonadoptees were at increased risk for mood disorders but the adoptive parents of bipolar adoptees were not at increased risk. These results showed that genetic—not adoptive—relationships mediated the familial risk for developing mood disorders.

Cadoret (1978) compared adoptees whose biological mothers had mood disorders with adoptees whose biological mothers did not have mood disorders. Among the adoptees there were no cases of bipolar disorder. However, the rate of unipolar disorder was much higher among adoptees with ill biological mothers compared with those having well biological mothers. However, because of the small sample size, the difference was not statistically significant so these results are difficult to interpret. In a later study, Cadoret, O'Gorman, Heywood, and Troughton (1985) showed that adoptees with a biological family history of mood disorder were more likely to have had an episode of illness compared with adoptees with no such family history. However, the difference was not statistically significant. In contrast, some environmental characteristics of the adoptive family were predictive of adoptee depression. These were alcohol use problems in the adoptive parents, other psychiatric illness in the adoptive parents, and death of the adoptive parent.

Wender *et al.* (1986) identified adult adoptees with mood disorders and control adoptees with no record of psychiatric illness. They matched the ill and control adoptees on demographic features of the adopting parents. Among relatives of ill adoptees, the risk to biological relatives was greater than the risk to adoptive relatives. Notably, the biological relatives of ill adoptees were six times more likely than the adoptive relatives to have completed suicide. The biological relatives had three times the rate of unipolar disorder and alcoholism compared with the adoptive relatives of ill adoptees.

In summary, the Danish study of Wender *et al.* confirmed the Belgian study by implicating genetic but not environmental relationships in the transmission of mood disorders. In contrast, the work of Cadoret *et al.* suggests a role for environmental mechanisms. Clearly, more work is needed to clarify these inconsistent findings.

MECHANISMS OF INHERITANCE OF MOOD DISORDERS

Segregation analysis examines the pattern of segregation of disorders in families and determines if this pattern is consistent with a hypothesized mode of transmission. In theory, such analyses can provide strong evidence for one mode of transmission (e.g., single major gene) over others (e.g., environmental transmission, polygenic inheritance).

Unfortunately, mathematical analyses of mood disorder pedigrees have not been able to support consistently a mode of genetic transmission for either unipolar or bipolar mood disorders. Reviews of segregation analysis studies find no strong support for either single gene or polygenic transmission, even when such factors as gender and polarity are taken into account in the analyses (Faraone *et al.*, 1990; Tsuang & Faraone, 1990; Moldin, Reich, & Rice 1991).

Linkage and Association Studies of Mood Disorders

Despite the failure of segregation analyses to confirm a specific mode of transmission, psychiatric geneticists turned to genetic linkage analyses to determine if genes influencing mood disorders could be discovered. This has led to much work and an equal amount of controversy. Although systematic searches of the genome have not produced strong evidence for linkage (Berrettini *et al.*, 1992; Detera-Wadleigh *et al.*, 1994), several regions of the genome have been implicated. However, because these findings have not been consistently replicated, they remain suggestive, not definitive.

X-Linkage. Prior to the discovery of DNA markers, several studies examined bipolar pedigrees informative for protan (red deficiency) or deutan (green deficiency) colorblindness, recessive X-linked traits with known chromosomal locations. Using these genetic markers, linkage between bipolar disorder and color blindness was suggested over two decades ago (Reich, Clayton, & Winokur, 1969; Winokur & Tanna, 1969; Mendlewicz, Fleiss, & Fieve, 1972). In fact, in one analysis, the odds favoring linkage were greater than 30,000 to 1 (Mendlewicz & Fleiss, 1974). Unfortunately, these early results were not easily replicated (Johnson & Leeman, 1977; Kidd et al., 1984) and, although some consistent results were reported (Baron, 1977; Baron et al., 1987), these were not supported in a follow-up study including additional DNA markers in the same pedigrees that had previously given evidence for X-linkage (Baron et al., 1993).

Gershon and colleagues (Gershon, Targum, Matthysse, & Bunney, 1979; Gershon et al., 1980) reported results from an international collaborative study of X-linkage under the auspices of the World Health Organization. This collaboration examined 16 pedigrees that had been ascertained through bipolar probands in the United States, Belgium, Switzerland, and Denmark. The overall evidence for linkage was equivocal, but separate analyses of subsamples strongly suggested the presence of significant heterogeneity. Based on 6 American pedigrees, close linkage could be definitively excluded. In contrast, the data from 8 Belgian pedigrees were more suggestive of linkage.

Additional positive studies of X-linkage have examined glucose-6-phosphate dehydrogenase (G6PD) deficiency and various DNA markers. All of these provide X-chromosome markers close to the locus for color-blindness. Of the three studies examining linkage with G6PD, one was clearly supportive and a second at least highly suggestive of X-chromosome involvement in affective disorders (Mendlewicz Linkowski, & Wilmotte, 1980; Del Zompo, Bocchetta, Goldin, & Corsini, 1984; Baron et al., 1987). Furthermore, one study using the F9 DNA marker was consistent with the presence of a bipolar gene on the X chromosome (Mendlewicz et al., 1987), but others using DNA markers in the same region have excluded linkage for bipolar (Berrettini et al., 1990) and unipolar (Neiswanger et al., 1990) disorders.

Taken together, the evidence from these studies is inconsistent with regard to X-linkage in bipolar-related affective disorders. Gershon and Bunney (1976) suggested that there might have been systematic procedural errors on the part of Mendlewicz and colleagues since most of the positive linkage results had come from this one group of investigators. Gershon (1991) demonstrated that the studies of Mendlewicz et al. from 1972 to 1975 do contain systematic genotyping errors because they show linkage to two markers at opposite ends of the X chromosome. He argued that the potential for systematic errors in these pedigrees diminishes their ability to support the hypothesis of X-linkage. Mendlewicz, Sandkvil, De Bruyn, and Van Broeckhoven (1991) pointed out that Gershon's conclusions do not apply to more recent reports of X-linkage. In contrast, Hebebrand (1992) pointed out that, despite some positive linkage findings, pedigrees showing characteristic features of X-linkage are rare.

Other Linkage and Association Results. Other genetic loci have shown some promise in linkage studies of mood disorders. The results for the HLA region of chromosome 6 were initially positive, with several sib-pair studies finding linkage and one pedigree study finding odds favoring linkage of 10^8 to 1 (Turner & Kins, 1983). However, as was the case for X-linkage, other studies reject linkage to this region (Tsuang & Faraone, 1990). Thus, further work is needed to confirm the positive findings.

Of 18 studies of HLA association in mood disorders, 8 found no evidence for an association. The others provided some evidence for an association but were inconsistent with one another because they implicated different HLA genes as associated with mood disorders (Tsuang & Faraone, 1990). These inconsistent results could be related to the fact that the reported investigations were performed in a variety of different countries with different ethnic groups. However, Tsuang and Faraone (1990) show that this is not the case. The most conservative interpretation of these results in that mood disorder is not associated with HLA. If such an association exists, it is either very weak or limited to a subset of patients.

In 1987 Egeland *et al.* reported significant evidence in favor of linkage for the HRAS1 locus on the short arm of chromosome 11. The original report was very compelling. The large pedigree collected from an old order Amish community provided a rare opportunity to detect linkage in a genetically homogeneous population. Also, the methodology was excellent. Unfortunately, although small positive LOD scores for this region have been reported (Lim *et al.*, 1993), most subsequent reports (Detera-Wadleigh *et al.*, 1987; Hodgkinson *et al.*, 1987; Gill, McKeon, & Humphries, 1988; Neiswanger *et al.*, 1990; Holmes *et al.*, 1991; Mendlewicz, Leboyer, *et al.*, 1991; Mitchell *et al.*, 1991) excluded linkage to this region and a follow-up study of Egeland and colleagues' pedigree cast doubt on the original finding (Kelsoe *et al.*, 1989). After additional diagnostic and genetic data were collected, the analyses excluded linkage to chromosome 11. This reversal was unexpected and may be related to genetic heterogeneity within the large pedigree. Alternatively, the original finding may have been a chance result.

On the other hand, there is some additional evidence suggesting that a gene in the HRAS1 region may be involved in bipolar disorder. Joffe, Horvath, and Tarvydas (1986) reported a family in which bipolar-related disorders and thalassemia minor appeared to cosegregate. Thalassemia minor is caused by mutation of a gene on the short arm of chromosome 11 close to the HRAS1 and INS loci. This region is of interest for association studies because it is close to the gene for tyrosine hydroxylase (TH). DNA markers at the TH locus were associated with bipolar disorder in a French sample (Leboyer et al., 1990), but no association was found in a British sample (Gill et al., 1991), two German samples (Korner, Fritze, & Propping, 1990; Lanczik et al., 1991) and a Japanese sample (Inayama et al., 1993). A small American sample initially suggested no association (Todd & O'Malley, 1989) but a larger series was consistent with an association between TH and bipolar disorder (Todd, O'Malley, Parsian, Simpson, & DePaulo, 1991). Also, a combined analysis of three European samples found a significant association between bipolar disorder and markers at the TH locus. Despite these findings, linkage between the TH locus and bipolar disorder has not been found (Byerley et al., 1992).

The long arm of chromosome 11 has also generated some interest. In an American pedigree reported by Smith et al., (1989), five members suffered from bipolar disorder and each had a translocation from chromosome 11 to chromosome 9. The translocation point on chromosome 11 was close to two genes that are relevant to psychiatric illness: the dopamine 2 receptor gene and the tyrosinase gene. Although it is reasonable to hypothesize that the illness in these families was caused by the translocation, subsequent attempts to detect linkage (Byerley et al., 1990; Holmes et al., 1991; Jensen et al., 1992; Mitchell et al., 1992; Nanko et al., 1994) and association (Korner et al., 1991; Nothen et al., 1992) to this region have not been successful.

A gene near the ABO region on chromosome 9 may play a role in bipolar disorder. Several studies have compared ABO blood groups between patients with mood disorders and healthy individuals. Nine of sixteen studies found a significant increase in blood type O; one reported a significant decrease of blood type O among mood disordered patients. Two studies found a significant increase in blood type B and one study found a significant increase in blood type A. Three studies found a significant decrease in blood type A (Tsuang & Faraone, 1990). The primary inference from these studies is the fairly strong suggestion that blood type O is found with greater frequency among patients with bipolar disorder than in individuals from the general population (Lavori, Keller, & Roth, 1984).

Unfortunately, the reported ABO associations are inconsistent with six of eight studies rejecting linkage to ABO (Tsuang & Faraone, 1990). Two studies were equivocal. The association and linkage results are difficult to reconcile. However, such a result would not be surprising if a gene of minor effect were located near the ABO locus (Plomin, 1990; Plomin, McClearn, Owen, & McGuffin, 1991). This is consistent with the finding that the gene for dopamine-β-hydroxylase (DBH) is strongly suspected to be closely linked to the ABO locus (Goldin et al., 1982; McKusick, 1986; Wilson, Elston, Siervogel, & Tran, 1988). Since DBH is critical to the synthesis of catecholamines, it is a reasonable candidate as an etiological gene for bipolar disorders.

Using the affected sibling-pair method, Berrettini *et al.* (1994) reported a potential linkage between bipolar disorder and marker loci near the centromere of chromosome 18. LOD scores were positive but not significant. In contrast, based on results of a nonparametric affected sib-pair analysis, Berrettini *et al.* concluded that chromosome 18 may harbor a gene of small effect that plays a role in the complex inheritance of bipolar disorder.

FUTURE DIRECTIONS

Family, twin, and adoption studies provide firm evidence that some mood disorders have a substantial genetic component. However, molecular genetic studies have not yet found the genes that underlie the inheritance of mood disorders. There have been many attempts to explain this situation as related to the clinical and epidemiological features of psychiatric disorders that point to complex inheritance—as opposed to single gene inheritance—for psychiatric disorders (Diehl & Kendler, 1989; Merikangas, Spence, & Kupfer, 1989; Elston & Wilson, 1990; Gershon, 1990; Green, 1990; Matthysse, 1990; Morton, 1990; Ott, 1990a,b; Risch, 1990; Suarez, Reich, Rice, & Cloninger, 1990; Weeks *et al.*, 1990; Spence *et al.*, 1992; Cloninger, 1994; Gershon & Cloninger, 1994).

Clearly, if mood disorders reflect the additive and/or epistatic (i.e., interactive) effects of several genes, then linkage to any single gene would be difficult to detect and, in some cases, extremely difficult to replicate (Suarez, Hampe, & Van Eerdewegh, 1994). Furthermore, assortative mating, genetic heterogeneity, sporadic cases, misclassification, and low penetrance may further complicate the picture. Although these problems can be overcome (Ott, 1991; Faraone & Santangelo, 1992; Faraone & Tsuang, 1994), to do so may require very large samples of well-characterized pedigrees.

Tsuang, Faraone, and Lyons (1993) noted that given the variable phenotypic expression of psychiatric genotypes, future genetic epidemiologic work should attempt to define more heritable phenotypes. They review several available methods including specific applications to mood disorders. For example, Rice and colleagues (Rice, Endicott, Knesevich, & Rochberg, 1987; Rice, Rochberg, Endicott, Lavori, & Miller, 1992) showed how an index of "caseness" (the degree to which an individual truly has a disorder) could be derived from diagnostic data collected at more than one time point. They reasoned that diagnoses that are stable over time are more likely to reflect a true underlying illness than diagnoses that are not stable. To define an index of caseness based on stability, they used clinical measures from patients with mood disorder diagnoses (e.g., number of symptoms, number of episodes) to predict who would and would not report a lifetime history of the disorder 6 years later. The result of this procedure is a logistic regression equation that uses the clinical measures to compute the probability that a case will be stable over a 6-year period. This probability is an index of caseness inasmuch as stability over time reflects the subject's true illness status.

For example, in their analysis of major depression, the caseness index ranged from a low of 0.46 for subjects having three symptoms and no history of treatment to 1.0 for those who had eight symptoms and a history of treatment (Rice *et al.*, 1992). These analyses confirmed an intuitive sense of how severity should be related to caseness and diagnostic stability.

In another approach to phenotype definition, Blacker and colleagues (Blacker, Lavori, Faraone, & Tsuang, 1993; Blacker & Tsuang, 1992, 1993) proposed comparing cases of depression observed in families of bipolar probands with cases of depression observed in families of depressed probands. Any feature that discriminated the two groups could be used in such comparisons. However, for the problem of bipolarity in depressed patients, these authors chose to focus on features shown by the phenomenology of depression in bipolar patients and in depressive patients who subsequently had a bipolar episode. They showed how logistic regression might be used to create a measure of caseness that indexed the probability that the depressed subject was a potential bipolar case.

For mood disorders, the problem of phenotype definition is complicated by their extensive comorbidity, and potential genetic relatedness to other disorders. A large literature suggests that anxiety disorders frequently co-occur with a major depressive disorder (Maser & Cloninger, 1990). This comorbidity has been reported for adults and children in both clinical and epidemiologic samples. Weissman, Prusoff, *et al.* (1984) reported an overall rate of anxiety disorders of 22% for children whose parents had a diagnosis of depression plus agoraphobia or panic disorder. In contrast, children of adults with depression only and children of normal controls had very low rates of anxiety disorders. Puig-Antich and Rabinovich (1986) found equally high rates of depression in the adult relatives of children with depression alone, depression with separation anxiety disorder (SAD), and SAD without depression. Last, Hersen, Kazdin, Francis, and Grubb (1987) reported very high rates of anxiety disorders and depression in the mothers of anxious children compared with mothers of controls. Livingston, Nugent, Rader, and Smith (1985) found elevated rates of depression in the relatives of children with anxiety disorders and in those with depression, but elevated rates of panic disorder were found only in the relatives of children with anxiety disorders and not in those with depression. These findings suggest that high rates of anxiety disorders in children of depressed parents are specifically associated with parental panic disorder or agoraphobia and not with depression.

The family genetic studies also suggest that the relationship between depression and anxiety is unidirectional. That is, parental anxiety disorder places children at risk for depression but parental depression does not place children at risk for anxiety disorders. It may be that depression that develops in anxious individuals may differ etiologically from depression that is not associated with anxiety. This is consistent with the finding that many patients with anxiety disorders subsequently experience onset of depression, but depressed patients do not usually develop an anxiety disorder (Cloninger, 1990). In addition, follow-up studies of adults have shown that individuals with depression without comorbid anxiety disorder seem to remain non-comorbid at follow-up, but cases characterized by a mixture of depressive and anxious symptoms seem to relapse with a mixture of the same symptoms. However, some studies have found that individuals with anxiety disorders but without comorbid depression rarely turn into pure depression cases at follow-up (Hagnell & Gräsbeck, 1990). Furthermore, Torgersen's (1990a,b) twin data show that depression confers a familial risk for panic disorder, depression, and the comorbid condition. In contrast, panic disorder alone is not familially linked to depression. These twin data have been interpreted as supporting the hypothesis that anxiety disorders with depression, and depression alone, may have the same etiologic factors while pure anxiety alone is another disorder. However, a large family study by Weissman *et al.* (1993) concluded that, although there was substantial comorbidity between panic disorder and major depression, the two were familially distinct disorders. In probands, panic disorder without depression increased the risk to relatives for panic disorder and panic with depression, but not depression alone. Similarly, depression without panic increased the risk to relatives for major depression and panic with depression, but not panic disorder alone.

Another disorder associated with mood disorders that may share genetic determinants is attention-deficit hyperactivity disorder (ADHD), a common disorder of childhood that also affects adults. As reviewed in detail elsewhere, converging evidence from family, twin, adoption, and segregation analysis studies suggests that genetic factors mediate the risk for ADHD (Faraone & Biederman, 1994a,b). There are high levels of comorbidity between ADHD and depression (Biederman, Faraone, Lapey, *et al.*, 1992; Angold & Costello, 1993; Biederman *et al.*, 1993) and many studies find high rates of major depression among the relatives of both depressed and nondepressed ADHD children (Stewart & Morrison, 1973; Welner, Welner, Stewart, Palkes, & Wish, 1977; Levy & Nurcombe, 1979; Mannuzza & Gittelman, 1984; Lahey et al., 1988; Schachar & Wachsmuth, 1990; Barkley, Fischer, Edlebrock, & Smallish, 1991; Bhatia, Nigam, Bohra, & Malik, 1991; Biederman, Faraone, Keenan, & Tsuang, 1991; Biederman, Faraone, Keenan, et al., 1992; Schachar, personal communication). Although the familial risk for depression is highest when the ADHD proband also exhibits antisocial behavior (Lahey et al., 1988; Barkley et al., 1991), it is still significant in families that are not selected through an antisocial proband (Faraone et al., 1995). This suggests that major depression is a nonspecific manifestation of the genetic susceptibility to ADHD (Biederman et al., 1991; Biederman, Faraone, Keenan, et al., 1992). This hypothesis predicts increased rates of ADHD in the children of depressed parents. Such increased rates have been reported in some family studies (Weissman, Prusoff, et al., 1984; Orvaschel, Walsh-Allis, & Ye, 1988; Welner & Rice, 1988; Grigoroiu-Serbanescu et al., 1991), but not others (Weissman et al., 1987). These conflicting results highlight the etiological complexities underlying psychiatric comorbidity and underscore the need for comorbidity assessments in studies of mood disorders.

The examples of anxiety disorders and ADHD illustrate the phenomenon of psychiatric comorbidity. Additional comorbid conditions that may share genetic causes with mood disorders include alcoholism (Merikangas, Weissman, Prusoff, Pauls, & Leckman, 1985; Merikangas, 1990; Winokur & Coryell, 1991; Coryell, Winokur, Keller, Scheftner, & Endicott, 1992; Kendler, Heath, Neale, Kessler, & Eaves, 1993; Maier, Lichtermann, & Minges, 1994; Merikangas, Risch, & Weissman, 1994), bulimia (Kendler et al., 1991; Walters et al., 1992), and migraine headache (Merikangas, Merikangas, & Angst, 1993).

SUMMARY

The risk for mood disorders increases with the proportion of genes shared with a mood-disordered patient. The risk to relatives is higher than the risk to the general population. It is also higher than the risk to relatives of well individuals as determined by double-blind case–control studies. Thus, family data unequivocally indicate that mood disorders are familial, i.e., they run in families.

The concordance rate for mood disorder among MZ twins is approximately three times the rate observed among DZ twins. This strongly suggests that genes play a crucial role in the familial transmission of these disorders. The MZ twin concordance rate is approximately 0.70 for bipolar disorder and 0.50 for unipolar disorder. Since concordance is not perfect, nonfamilial environmental factors must play a role in the etiology of mood disorders. These factors appear to be less prominent for bipolar than for unipolar disorder. The conclusions from the twin studies agree with two methodologically strong adoption studies indicating biological relationships to be better predictors for the risk of mood disorders than are adoptive relationships. That is, both types of study suggest that the familial transmission of these disorders has a primarily genetic source. The environmental factors that cause illness are likely to be nonfamilial. However, since the adoption study literature contains some conflicting reports, we need more adoption studies to provide convergent support for these assertions.

The genetic relationship between unipolar and bipolar disorders is poorly understood. Further research into this area must distinguish recurrent unipolar cases that are not likely to have a subsequent manic episode from nonrecurrent cases that may be bipolar. It is probably true that cases of unipolar disorder within families that manifest bipolar disorder are genetic variants of bipolar disorder. The clearest and most consistent difference between the two forms of mood disorder is that relatives of bipolar probands are at a greater risk for both unipolar and bipolar disorders than are relatives of unipolar probands. Evidence from both family and twin studies supports this conclusion. Thus, it is likely that bipolar disorder has a greater familial component than does unipolar disorder; unipolar appears to be more greatly affected by nonfamilial, environmental factors.

Despite strong evidence for a genetic component to mood disorders, mathematical modeling studies do not consistently support a specific mode of genetic transmission. Also, linkage and association studies have led to equivocal results. Since mathematical modeling and linkage analyses have tested relatively simple models of genetic transmission, it may be that more complex models are needed to describe the transmission of mood disorders or that advances in nosology are needed to define genetic variants of these disorders. Future linkage work should consider ascertaining large samples of well-characterized pedigrees that will be suitable for finding genes under conditions of complex inheritance.

ACKNOWLEDGMENTS

Preparation of this chapter was supported in part by the Veterans Administration's Medical Research and Health Services Research and Development Programs and National Institute of Mental Health Grants 1 R01MH41879-01, 5 UO1 MH46318-02, and R37MH43518-01.

REFERENCES

American Psychiatric Association. (1994). *Diagnostic and statistical manual of mental disorders* (4th ed.). Washington, DC: American Psychiatric Association.

Andreasen, N. C., Rice, J., Endicott, J., Coryell, W., Grove, W. M., & Reich, T. (1987). Familial rates of affective disorder. A report from the National Institute of Mental Health collaborative study. *Archives of General Psychiatry 44,* 461–469.

Angold, A., & Costello, E. J. (1993). Depressive comorbidity in children and adolescents: Empirical, theoretical, and methodological issues. *American Journal of Psychiatry, 150,* 1779–1791.

Barkley, R. A., Fischer, M., Edlebrock, C., & Smallish, L. (1991). The adolescent outcome of hyperactive children diagnosed by research criteria: III. Mother–child interactions, family conflicts and maternal psychopathology. *Journal of Child Psychology and Psychiatry, 32,* 233–255.

Baron, M. (1977). Linkage between an X-chromosome marker (deutan color blindness) and bipolar affective illness: Occurrence in the family of a lithium carbonate-responsive schizoaffective proband. *Archives of General Psychiatry, 34,* 721–725.

Baron, M., Freimer, N. F., Risch, N., Lerer, B., Alexander, J. R., Straub, R. E., Asokan, S., Das, K., Peterson, A., Amos, J., Endicott, J., Ott, J., & Gilliam, T. C. (1993). Diminished support for linkage between manic depressive illness and X-chromosome markers in three Israeli pedigrees. *Nature Genetics, 3,* 49–55.

Baron, M., Risch, N., Hamburger, R., Mandel, B., Kushner, S., Newman, M., Drumer, D., & Belmaker, R. H. (1987). Genetic linkage between X-chromosome markers and bipolar affective illness, *Nature, 326,* 289–292.

Berrettini, W. H., Detera-Wadleigh, S. D., Goldin, L. R., Martinez, M., Hsieh, W.-T., Hoehe, M., Choi, H., Muniec, D., Ferraro, T. N., Guroff, J. G., Kazuba, D., Harris, N., Kron, E., Nurnberger, J. I., Jr., Alexander, R. C., & Gershon, E. S. (1992). Genomic screening for genes predisposing to bipolar disease. *Psychiatry Genetics, 2,* 191–208.

Berrettini, W. H., Ferraro, T. N., Goldin, L. R., Weeks, D. E., Detera-Wadleigh, S., Nurnberger, J. I., Jr., & Gershon, E. S. (1994). Chromosome 18 DNA markers and manic-depressive illness: Evidence for a susceptibility gene. *Proceedings of the National Academy of Sciences USA, 91,* 5918–5921.

Berrettini, W. H., Goldin, L. R., Gelernter, J., Gejman, P. V., Gershon, E. S., & Detera-Wadleigh, S. (1990). X-chromosome markers and manic-depressive illness. Rejection of linkage to Xq28 in nine bipolar pedigrees. *Archives of General Psychiatry, 47,* 366–373.

Bertelsen, A., Harvald, B., & Hauge, M. (1977). A Danish twin study of manic-depressive disorders. *British Journal of Psychiatry, 130,* 330–351.

Bhatia, M., Nigam, V., Bohra, N., & Malik, S. (1991). Attention deficit disorder with hyperactivity among paediatric outpatients. *Journal of Child Psychology and Psychiatry, 32,* 297–306.

Biederman, J., Faraone, S. V., Keenan, K., Benjamin, J., Krifcher, B., Moore, C., Sprich-Bukminister, S., Ugaglia, K., Jellinek, M. S., Steingard, R., Spencer, T., Norman, D., Kolodny, R., Kraus, I., Perrin, J., Keller, M. B., & Tsuang, M. T. (1992). Further evidence for family-genetic risk factors in attention deficit hyperactivity disorder. Patterns of comorbidity in probands and relatives in psychiatrically and pediatrically referred samples. *Archives of General Psychiatry, 49,* 728–738.

Biederman, J., Faraone, S. V., Keenan, K., & Tsuang, M. T. (1991). Evidence of familial association between attention deficit disorder and major affective disorders. *Archives of General Psychiatry, 48,* 633–642.

Biederman, J., Faraone, S. V., & Lapey, K. (1992). Comorbidity of diagnosis in attention deficit hyperactivity disorder (ADHD). *Child and Adolescent Psychiatric Clinics of North America, 1,* 335–360.

Biederman, J., Faraone, S. V., Spencer, T., Wilens, T., Norman, D., Lapey, K. A., Mick, E., Lehman, B. K., & Doyle, A. (1993). Patterns of psychiatric comorbidity, cognition, and psychosocial functioning in adults with attention deficit hyperactivity disorder. *American Journal of Psychiatry, 150,* 1792–1798.

Blacker, D., Lavori, P. W., Faraone, S. V., & Tsuang, M. T. (1993). Unipolar relatives in bipolar pedigrees: A search for indicators underlying bipolarity. *American Journal of Medical Genetics, Neuropsychiatric Genetics, 48,* 192–199.

Blacker, D., & Tsuang, M. T. (1992). Contested boundaries of bipolar disorder and the limits of categorical diagnosis in psychiatry. *American Journal of Psychiatry, 149,* 1473–1483.

Blacker, D., & Tsuang, M. T. (1993). Unipolar relatives in bipolar pedigrees: Are they bipolar? *Psychiatric Genetics, 3,* 5–16.

Blazer, D. G., Kessler, R. C., McGonagle, K. A., & Swartz, M. S. (1994). The prevalence and distribution of major depression in a national community sample: The national comorbidity survey. *American Journal of Psychiatry, 151,* 979–986.

Boyd, J. H., Burke, J. D., Gruenberg, E., Holzer, C. E., Rae, D. S., George, L. K., Karno, M., Stoltzman, R., McEvoy, L., & Nestadt, G. (1984). Exclusion criteria of DSM-III. A study of co-occurrence of hierarchy-free syndromes. *Archives of General Psychiatry, 41,* 983–989.

Byerley, W., Leppert, M., O'Connell, P., Mellon, C., Holik, J., Lubbers, A., Reimherr, F., Jenson, S., Hill, K., Wender, P., Grandy, D., Litt, M., Lalouel, J.-M., Civelli, O., & White, R. (1990). D$_2$ dopamine receptor gene not linked to manic-depression in three families. *Psychiatric Genetics, 1,* 55–62.

Byerley, W., Plaetke, R., Hoff., M., Jensen, S., Holik, J., Reimherr, F., Mellon, C., Wender, P., O'Connell, P., & Leppert, M. (1992). Tyrosine hydroxylase gene not linked to manic-depression in seven of eight pedigrees. *Human Heredity, 42,* 259–263.

Cadoret, R. J. (1978). Evidence for genetic inheritance of primary affective disorder in adoptees. *American Journal of Psychiatry, 135,* 463–466.

Cadoret, R. J., O'Gorman, T. W., Heywood, E., & Troughton, E. (1985). Genetic and environmental factors in major depression. *Journal of Affective Disorders, 9,* 155–164.

Cloninger, C. R. (1990). Comorbidity of anxiety and depression. *Journal of Clinical Psychopharmacology, 10,* 43S–46S.

Cloninger, C. R. (1994). Turning point in the design of linkage studies of schizophrenia. *American Journal of Medical Genetics, Neuropsychiatric Genetics, 54,* 83–92.

Coryell, W., Winokur, G., Keller, M., Scheftner, W., & Endicott, J. (1992). Alcoholism and primary major depression: A family study approach to co-existing disorders. *Journal of Affective Disorders, 24,* 93–99.

Del Zompo, M., Bocchetta, A., Goldin, L. R., & Corsini, G. U. (1984). Linkage between X-chromosome markers and manic-depressive illness. *Acta Psychiatrica Scandinavica, 70,* 282–287.

Detera-Wadleigh, S. D., Berrettini, W. H., Goldin, L. R., Boorman, D., Anderson, S., & Gershon, E. S. (1987). Close linkage of c-Harvey-ras-1 and the insulin gene to affective disorder is ruled out in three North American pedigrees. *Nature, 325,* 806–808.

Detera-Wadleigh, S. D., Hsieh, W.-T., Berrettini, W. H., Goldin, L. R., Rollins, D. Y., Muniec, D., Grewal, R., Guroff, J. J., Turner, G., Coffman, D., Barrick, J., Mills, K., Murray, J., Donohue, S. J., Klein, D. C., Sanders, J., Nurnberger, J. I., Jr., & Gershon, E. S. (1994). Genetic linkage mapping for a susceptibility locus to bipolar illness: Chromosomes 2, 3, 4, 7, 9, 10p, 11p, 22, and Xpter. *American Journal of Medical Genetics (Neuropsychiatric Genetics), 54,* 206–218.

Diehl, S. R., & Kendler, K. S. (1989). Strategies for linkage studies of schizophrenia: Pedigrees, DNA markers, and statistical analyses. *Schizophrenia Bulletin, 15,* 403–419.

Egeland, J. A., Gerhard, D. S., Pauls, D. L., Sussex, J. N., Kidd, K. K., Allen, C. R., Hostetter, A. M., & Housman, D. E. (1987). Bipolar affective disorders linked to DNA markers on chromosome 11. *Nature, 325,* 783–787.

Elston, R. C., & Wilson, A. F. (1990). Genetic linkage and complex diseases: A comment. *Genetic Epidemiology, 7,* 17–19.

Endicott, J., Nee, J., Andreasen, N., Clayton, P., Keller, M., & Coryell, W. (1985). Bipolar II: Combine or keep separate? *Journal of Affective Disorders, 8,* 17–28.

Faraone, S., & Biederman, J. (1994a). Genetics of attention-deficit hyperactivity disorder. *Child and Adolescent Psychiatric Clinics of North America, 3,* 285–302.

Faraone, S., & Biederman, J. (1994b). Is attention deficit hyperactivity disorder familial? *Harvard Review of Psychiatry, 1,* 271–287.

Faraone, S. V., Biederman, J., Chen, W. J., Milberger, S., Warburton, R. M., & Tsuang, M. T. (1995). Genetic heterogeneity in attention deficit hyperactivity disorder: Gender, psychiatric comorbidity and parental illness. *Journal of Abnormal Psychology, 104,* 334–345.

Faraone, S. V., Kremen, W. S., & Tsuang, M. T. (1990). Genetic transmission of major affective disorders: Quantitative models and linkage analyses. *Psychological Bulletin, 108,* 109–127.

Faraone, S. V., & Santangelo, S. (1992). Methods in genetic epidemiology. In M. Fava & J. F. Rosenbaum (Eds.), *Research designs and methods in psychiatry.* Amsterdam: Elsevier.

Faraone, S. V., & Tsuang, M. T. (1994). Methods in psychiatric genetics. In M. Tohen, M. T. Tsuang, G. E. P. Zahner (Eds.), *Textbook in psychiatric epidemiology.* New York: Wiley.

Feighner, J. P., Robins, E., Guze, S. B., *et al.* (1972). Diagnostic criteria for use in psychiatric research. *Archives of General Psychiatry, 26,* 57–63.

Gershon, E. S. (1990). Genetic linkage and complex disease: A comment. *Genetic Epidemiology, 7,* 21–23.

Gershon, E. S. (1991). Marker genotyping errors in old data on X-linkage in bipolar illness. *Biological Psychiatry, 29,* 721–729.

Gershon, E. S., & Bunney, W. E., Jr. (1976). The question of X-linkage in bipolar manic-depressive illness. *Journal of Psychiatric Research, 13,* 99–117.

Gershon, E. S., & Cloninger, C. R. (1994). *Genetic approaches to mental disorders.* Washington, DC: American Psychiatric Press.

Gershon, E. S., Hamovit, J., Guroff, J. J., Dibble, E., Leckman, J. F., Sceery, W., Targum, S. D., Nurnberger, J. I., Jr., Goldin, L. R., & Bunney, W. E., Jr. (1982). A family study of schizoaffective, bipolar I, bipolar II, unipolar and normal control probands. *Archives of General Psychiatry, 39,* 1157–1167.

Gershon, E. S., Mark, A., Cohen, N., Belizon, N., Baron, M., & Knobe, K. E. (1975). Transmitted factors in the morbid risk of affective disorders: A controlled study. *Journal of Psychiatric Research, 12,* 283–299.

Gershon, E. S., Mendlewicz, J., Gastpar, M., Bech, P., Goldin, L. R., Kielholz, P., Rafaelsen, O. J., Vartanian, F., & Bunney, W. E., Jr. (1980). A collaborative study of genetic linkage of bipolar manic-depressive illness and red/green colorblindness. *Acta Pschiatrica Scandinavica, 61,* 319–338.

Gershon, E. S., Targum, S. D., Matthysse, S., & Bunney, W. E., Jr., (1979). Color blindness not closely linked to bipolar illness: Report of a new pedigree series. *Archives of General Psychiatry, 36,* 1423–1430.

Gill, M., Castle, D., Hunt, N., Clements, A., Sham, P., & Murray, R. M. (1991). Tyrosine hydroxylase polymorphisms and bipolar affective disorder. *Journal of Psychiatric Research, 25,* 179–184.

Gill, M., McKeon, P., & Humphries, T. (1988). Linkage analysis of manic depression in an Irish family using H-ras 1 and INS DNA markers. *Journal of Medical Genetics, 25,* 634–637.

Goldin, L. R., Gershon, E. S., Lake, C. R., Murphy, D. L., McGinniss, M., & Sparkes, R. S. (1982). Segregation and linkage studies of plasma dopamine-beta-hydroxylase (DBH), erythrocyte catechol-O-methyltransferase (COMT), and platelet monoamine oxidase (MAO): Possible linkage between the ABO locus and a gene controlling DBH activity. *American Journal of Human Genetics, 34,* 250–262.

Green, P. (1990). Genetic linkage and complex diseases: A comment. *Genetic Epidemiology, 7,* 25–27.

Grigoroiu-Serbanescu, M., Christodorescu, D., Magureanu, S., Jipescu, I., Totoescu, A., Marinescu, E., Ardelean, V., & Popa, S. (1991). Adolescent offspring of endogenous unipolar depressive parents and of normal parents. *Journal of Affective Disorders, 21,* 185–198.

Hagnell, O., & Gräsbeck, A. (1990). Comorbidity of anxiety and depression in the Lundby 25-year prospective study: The pattern of subsequent episodes. In *Comorbidity of mood and anxiety disorders* (pp. 139–152). Washington, DC: American Psychiatric Press.

Hebebrand, J. (1992). A critical appraisal of X-linked bipolar illness evidence for the assumed mode of inheritance is lacking. *British Journal of Psychiatry, 160,* 7–11.

Hodgkinson, S., Sherrington, R., Gurling, H., Marchbanks, R., Reeders, S., Mallet, J., McInnis, M., Petursson, H., & Brynjolfsson, J. (1987). Molecular genetic evidence for heterogeneity in manic depression. *Nature, 325,* 805–806.

Holmes, D., Brynjolfsson, J., Brett, P., Curtis, D., Petursson, H., Sherrington, R., & Gurling, H. (1991). No evidence for a susceptibility locus predisposing to manic depression in the region of the dopamine (D2) receptor gene. *British Journal of Psychiatry, 158,* 635–641.

Inayama, Y., Yoneda, H., Sakai, T., Ishida, T., Kobayashi, S.-I., Nonomura, Y., Kono, Y., Koh, J., & Asaba, H. (1993). Lack of association between bipolar affective disorder and tyrosine hydroxylase DNA marker. *American Journal of Medical Genetics, Neuropsychiatric Genetics, 48,* 87–89.

Jensen, S., Plaetke, R., Holik, J., Hoff, M., O'Connell, P., Reimherr, F., Wender, P., Zhou, Q. Y., Civelli, O., Litt, M., Leppert, M., & Byerley, W. (1992). Linkage analysis of the D1 dopamine receptor gene and manic depression in six families. *Human Heredity, 42,* 269–275.

Joffe, R. T., Horvath, Z., & Tarvydas, I. (1986). Bipolar affective disorder and thalassemia minor. *American Journal of Psychiatry, 143,* 933.

Johnson, G. F. S., & Leeman, M. M. (1977). Analysis of familial factors in bipolar affective illness. *Archives of General Psychiatry, 34,* 1074–1083.

Kelsoe, J. R., Ginns, E. I., Egeland, J. A., Gerhard, D. S., Goldstein, A. M., Bale, S. J., Pauls, D. L., Long, R. T., Kidd, K. K., Conte, G., Housman, D. E., & Paul, S. M. (1989). Re-evaluation of the linkage relationship between chromosome 11p loci and the gene for bipolar affective disorder in the old order Amish. *Nature, 342,* 238–243.

Kendler, K. S., Heath, A. C., Neale, M. C., Kessler, R. C., & Eaves, L. J. (1993). Alcoholism and major depression in women. A twin study of the causes of comorbidity. *Archives of General Psychiatry, 50,* 690–698.

Kendler, K. S., Kessler, R. C., Neale, M. C., Heath, A. C., & Eaves, L. J. (1993). The prediction of major depression in women: Toward an integrated etiologic model. *American Journal of Psychiatry, 150,* 1139–1148.

Kendler, K. S., MacLean, C., Neale, M., Kessler, R., Heath, A., & Eaves, L. (1991). The genetic epidemiology of bulimia nervosa. *American Journal of Psychiatry, 148,* 1627–1637.

Kendler, K. S., Neale, M. C., Kessler, R. C., Heath, A. C., & Eaves, L. J. (1992). A population-based twin study of major depression in women. The impact of varying definitions of illness. *Archives of General Psychiatry, 49,* 257–266.

Kendler, K. S., Neale, M. C., Kessler, R. C., Heath, A. C., & Eaves, L. J. (1993). A longitudinal twin study of 1-year prevalence of major depression in women. *Archives of General Psychiatry, 50,* 843–852.

Kendler, K. S., Pedersen, N., Johnson, L., Neale, M. C., & Mathe, A. A. (1993). A pilot Swedish twin study of affective illness, including hospital- and population-ascertained subsamples. *Archives General Psychiatry, 50,* 699–706.

Kessler, R. C., McGonagle, K. A., Zhao, S., Nelson, C. B., Hughes, M., Eshlerman, S., Wittchen, H.-U., & Kendler, K. S. (1994). Lifetime and 12-month prevalence of DSM-III-R psychiatric disorders in the United States. Results from the national comorbidity survey. *Archives of General Psychiatry, 51,* 8–19.

Kidd, K. K., Egeland, J. A., Molthan, L., Pauls, D. L., Kruger, S. D., & Messner, K. H. (1984). Amish study: IV. Genetic linkage study of pedigrees of bipolar probands. *American Journal of Psychiatry, 141,* 1042–1048.

Korner, J., Fritz, J., & Propping, P. (1990). RFLP alleles at the tyrosine hydroxylase locus: No association found to affective disorders. *Psychiatric Research, 32,* 275–280.

Korner, J., Nothen, M., Erdmann, J., Cichon, S., Lanczik, M., Fritze, J., Moller, H-.J., & Propping, P. (1991). RFLPS at the loci for dopamine D1 and D2 receptors: An association study in bipolar affective disorder and schizophrenia. *Psychiatric Genetics, 2,* 83.

Lahey, B. B., Piacentini, J. C., McBurnett, K., Stone, P., Hartdagen, S., & Hynd, G. (1988). Psychopathology in parents of children with conduct disorder and hyperactivity. *Journal of the American Academy of Child and Adolescent Psychiatry, 27,* 163–170.

Lanczik, M., Nothen, M., Erdmann, J., Cichon, S., Korner, J., Fritze, J., Mallet, J., Moller, H.-J., & Propping, P. (1991). RFLP alleles at the tyrosine hydroxylase locus in schizophrenic and healthy control probands. *Psychiatric Genetics, 2,* 84.

Last, C. G., Hersen, M., Kazdin, A. E., Francis, G., & Grugg, H. J. (1987). Psychiatric illness in the mothers of anxious children. *American Journal of Psychiatry, 144,* 1580–1583.

Lavori, P. W., Keller, M. B., & Roth, S. L. (1984). Affective disorders and ABO blood groups: New data and a reanalysis of the literature using the logistic transformation of proportions. *Journal of Psychiatric Research, 18,* 119–129.

Leboyer, M., Malafosse, A., Boularand, S., Campion, D., Gheysen, F., Samolyk, D., Henriksson, B., Denise, E., Des Lauriers, A., Lepine, J.-P., Zarifian, E., Clerget-Darpoux, F., & Mallet, J. (1990). Tyrosine hydroxylase polymorphisms associated with manic-depressive illness. *Lancet, 335,* 1219.

Levy, F., & Nurcombe, B. (1979). Depression and anxiety in the mothers of hyperactive children. In J. Mendlewicz & B. Shopsin (Eds.), *Genetic aspects of affective illness: Current concepts.* New York: Luce Publications.

Lim, L. C. C., Gurling, H., Curtis, D., Brynjolfsson, J., Petursson, H., & Gill, M. (1993). Linkage between tyrosine hydroxylase gene and affective disorder cannot be excluded in two of six pedigrees. *American Journal of Medical Genetics, Neuropsychiatric Genetics, 48,* 223–228.

Livingston, R., Nugent, H., Rader, L., & Smith, G. R. (1985). Family histories of depressed and severely anxious children. *American Journal of Psychiatry, 142,* 1497–1499.

McGuffin, P., Katz, R., & Rutherford, J. (1991). Nature nurture and depression: A twin study. *Psychological Medicine, 21,* 329–335.

McKusick, V. (1986). *Mendelian inheritance in man.* Baltimore: Johns Hopkins University Press.

Maier, W., Lichtermann, D., & Minges, J. (1994). The relationship between alcoholism and unipolar depression. A controlled family study. *Journal of Psychiatric Research, 28,* 303–317.

Mannuzza, S., & Gittelman, R. (1984). The adolescent outcome of hyperactive girls. *Psychiatric Research, 13,* 19–29.

106 MING T. TSUANG and STEPHEN V. FARAONE

Marneros, A., & Tsuang, M. T. (1986). *Schizoaffective psychoses*. Berlin: Springer-Verlag.
Maser, J. D., & Cloninger, C. R. (1990). *Comorbidity of mood and anxiety disorders*. Washington, DC: American Psychiatric Press.
Matthysse, S. (1990). Genetic linkage and complex diseases: A comment. *Genetic Epidemiology, 7,* 29–31.
Mendlewicz, J., & Fleiss, J. L. (1974). Linkage studies with X-chromosome markers in bipolar (manic-depressive) and unipolar (depressive) illness. *Biological Psychiatry, 9,* 261–294.
Mendlewicz, J., Fleiss, J. L., & Fieve, R. R. (1972). Evidence for X-linkage in the transmission of manic-depressive illness. *Journal of the American Medical Association, 222,* 1624–1627.
Mendlewicz, J., Leboyer, M., De Bruyn, A., Malfosse, A., Sevy, S., Hirsch, D., Van Broeckhoven, C., & Mallet, J. (1991). Absence of linkage between chromosome 11p15 markers and manic-depressive illness in a Belgian pedigree. *American Journal of Psychiatry, 148,* 1683–1687.
Mendlewicz, J., Linkowski, P., & Wilmotte, J. (1980). Linkage between glucose-6-phosphate dehydrogenase deficiency and manic-depressive psychosis. *British Journal of Psychiatry, 137,* 337–342.
Mendlewicz, J., & Rainer, J. D. (1977). Adoption study supporting genetic transmission in manic-depressive illness. *Nature, 268,* 327–329.
Mendlewicz, J., Sandkuil, L. A., De Bruyn, A., & Van Broeckhoven, C. (1991). X-linkage in bipolar illness. *Biological Psychiatry, 29,* 730–734.
Mendlewicz, J., Simon, P., Sezy, S., Charon, F., Brocas, H., Legros, S., & Vassart, G. (1987). Polymorphic DNA marker on X-chromosome and manic depression. *Lancet, 1,* 1230–1232.
Merikangas, K. R. (1990). The genetic epidemiology of alcoholism. *Psychological Medicine, 20,* 11–22.
Merikangas, K. R., Merikangas, J. R., & Angst, J. (1993). Headache syndromes and psychiatric disorders: Association and familial transmission. *Journal of Psychiatric Research, 1993, 2.*
Merikangas, K. R., Risch, N. J., & Weissman, M. M. (1994). Comorbidity and cotransmission of alcoholism, anxiety and depression. *Psychological Medicine, 24,* 69–80.
Merikangas, K. R., Spence, A., & Kupfer, D. J. (1989). Linkage studies of bipolar disorder: Methodologic and analytic issues. Report of MacArthur Foundation workshop on linkage and clinical features in affective disorders. *Archives General Psychiatry, 46,* 1137–1141.
Merikangas, K. R., Weissman, M. M., Prusoff, B. A., Pauls, D. L., & Leckman, J. F. (1985). Depressives with secondary alcoholism: Psychiatric disorders in offspring. *Journal Studies of Alcohol, 46,* 199–204.
Mitchell, P., Selbie, L., Waters, B., Donald, J., Vivero, C., Tully, M., & Shine, J. (1992). Exclusion of close linkage of bipolar disorder to dopamine D_1 and D_2 receptor gene markers. *Journal of Affective Disorders, 25,* 1–12.
Mitchell, P., Waters, B., Morrison, N., Shine, J., Donald, J., & Eisman, J. (1991). Close linkage of bipolar disorder to chromosome 11 markers is excluded in two large Australian pedigrees. *Journal of Affective Disorders, 21,* 23–32.
Moldin, S. O., Reich, T., & Rice, J. P. (1991). Current perspectives on the genetics of unipolar depression. *Behavioral Genetics, 21,* 211–242.
Morton, N. E. (1990). Genetic linkage and complex diseases: A comment. *Genetic Epidemiology, 7,* 33–34.
Nanko, S., Fukuda, R., Hattori, M., Sasaki, T., Dai, X. Y., Kanba, S., Kato, T., & Kazamatsuri, H. (1994). Linkage studies between affective disorder and dopamine D_2, D_3, and D_4 receptor gene loci in four Japanese pedigrees. *Psychiatric Research, 52,* 149–157.
Neiswanger, K., Slaugenhaupt, S. A., Hughes, H. B., Frank, E., Frankel, D. R., McCarty,

M. J., Chakravarti, A., Zubenko, G. S., Kupfer, D. J., & Kaplan, B. B. (1990). Evidence against close linkage of unipolar affective illness to human chromosome 11p markers HRAS1 and INS and chromosome Xq marker DXS52. *Biological Psychiatry, 28,* 63–72.

Nothen, M. M., Erdmann, J., Korner, J., Lanczik, M., Fritzer, J., Fimmers, R., Grandy, D. K., O'Dowd, B., & Propping, P. (1992). Lack of association between dopamine D_1 and D_2 receptor genes and bipolar affective disorder. *American Journal of Psychiatry, 149,* 199–201.

Orvaschel, H., Walsh-Allis, G., & Ye, W. (1988). Psychopathology in children of parents with recurrent depression. *Journal of Abnormal Psychology, 16,* 17–28.

Ott, J. (1990a). Genetic linkage and complex diseases: A comment. *Genetic Epidemiology, 7,* 35–36.

Ott, J. (1990b). Invited editorial: Cutting a Gordian knot in the linkage analysis of complex human traits. *American Journal of Human Genetics, 46,* 219–221.

Ott, J. (1991). *Analysis of human genetic linkage.* Baltimore: Johns Hopkins University Press.

Plomin, R. (1990). The role of inheritance in behavior. *Science, 248,* 183–188.

Plomin, R., McClearn, G. E., Owen, M., & McGuffin, P. (1991). Quantitative genetics, molecular genetics, and dimensions of normal variation. *Behavior and Brain Science,* February 28th.

Puig-Antich, J., & Rabinovich, H. (1986). Relationship between affective and anxiety disorders in childhood. In R. Gittelman (Ed.), *Anxiety disorders of childhood* (pp. 136–156). New York: Guilford Press.

Reich, T., Clayton, P. J., & Winokur, G. (1969). Family history studies: V. The genetics of mania. *American Journal of Psychiatry, 125,* 64–75.

Rice, J. P., Endicott, J., Knesevich, M. A., & Rochberg, N. (1987). The estimation of diagnostic sensitivity using stability data: An application to major depressive disorder. *Journal of Psychiatric Research, 21,* 337–345.

Rice, J. P., Rochberg, N., Endicott, J., Lavori, P. W., & Miller, C. (1992). Stability of psychiatric diagnoses. An application to the affective disorders. *Archives of General Psychiatry, 49,* 824–830.

Risch, N. (1990). Genetic linkage and complex diseases, with special reference to psychiatric disorders. *Genetic Epidemiology, 7,* 3–7.

Sadovnick, A. D., Remick, R. A., Lam, R., Zis, A. P., Yee, I. M. L., Huggins, M. J., & Baird, P. A. (1994). Mood disorder service genetic database: Morbidity risks for mood disorders in 3,942 first-degree relatives of 671 index cases with single depression, recurrent depression, bipolar I, or bipolar II. *American Journal of Medical Genetics, Neuropsychiatric Genetics, 54,* 132–140.

Schachar, R., & Wachsmuth, R. (1990). Hyperactivity and parental psychopathology. *Journal of Child Psychology Psychiatry, 31,* 381–392.

Smith, M., Wasmuth, J., McPherson, J. D., Wagner, C., Grandy, D., Civelli, O., Potkin, S., & Litt, M. (1989). Cosegregation of an 11q22.3–9.22 translocation with affective disorder: Proximity of the dopamine D_2 receptor relative to the translocation breakpoint. *American Journal of Human Genetics, 45,* A220.

Spence, M. A., Bishop, D. T., Boehnke, M., Elston, R. C., Falk, C., Hodge, S. E., Ott, J., Rice, J., Merikangas, K., & Kupfer, D. (1992). Methodological issues in linkage analyses for psychiatric disorders: Secular trends, assortative mating, bilineal pedigrees. Report of the MacArthur Foundation Network I Task Force on Methodological Issues. *Human Heredity.*

Spitzer, R. L., Endicott, J., & Robins. E. (1978). Research diagnostic criteria: Rationale and reliability. *Archives of General Psychiatry, 35,* 773–782.

Stewart, M. A., & Morrison, J. R. (1973). Affective disorders among the relatives of hyperactive children. *Journal of Child Psychology and Psychiatry, 14,* 209–212.

Suarez, B. K., Hampe, C. L., & Van Eerdewegh, P. (1994). Problems of replicating linkage claims in psychiatry. In E. S. Gershon, C. R. Cloninger, & J. E. Barrett (Eds.), *Genetic approaches in mental disorders* (pp. 23–46). Washington, DC: American Psychiatric Press.

Suarez, B. K., Reich, T., Rice, J. P., & Cloninger, C. R. (1990). Genetic linkage and complex diseases: A comment. *Genetic Epidemiology, 7,* 37–40.

Todd, R. D., & O'Malley, K. L. (1989). Population frequencies of tyrosine hydroxylase restriction fragment length polymorphisms in bipolar affective disorder. *Biological Psychiatry, 25,* 626–630.

Todd, R. D., O'Malley, K. L. Parsian, A., Simpson, S. G., & DePaulo, J. R. (1991). Bipolar affective disorder and alleles of the tyrosine hydroxylase locus. *Psychiatric Genetics, 2,* 47.

Torgersen, S. (1990a). Comorbidity of major depression and anxiety disorders in twin pairs. *American Journal of Psychiatry, 147,* 1199–1202.

Torgersen, S. (1990b). A twin-study perspective of the comorbidity of anxiety and depression. In Cloninger (Ed.), *Comorbidity of mood and anxiety disorders* (pp. 367–378). Washington, DC: American Psychiatric Press.

Tsuang, M. T., & Faraone, S. V. (1990). *The genetics of mood disorders.* Baltimore: Johns Hopkins University Press.

Tsuang, M. T., & Faraone, S. V. (1994). Schizophrenia. In G. Winokur & P. Clayton (Eds.), *Medical basis of psychiatry* (2nd ed., pp. 87–114). Philadelphia: Saunders.

Tsuang, M. T., Faraone, S. V., & Lyons, M. J. (1993). Identification of the phenotype in psychiatric genetics. *European Archives of Psychiatry and Neurologic Science, 682,* 1–12.

Tsuang, M. T., Winokur, G., & Crowe, R. R. (1980). Morbidity risks of schizophrenia and affective disorders among first-degree relatives of patients with schizophrenia, mania, depression and surgical conditions. *British Journal of Psychiatry, 137,* 497–504.

Turner, W. J., & Kins, G. (1983). BPD2 an autosomal dominant form of bipolar affective disorder. *Biological Psychiatry, 18,* 63–87.

Walters, E. E., Neale, M. C., Eaves, L. J., Heath, A. C., Kessler, R. C., & Kendler, K. S. (1992). Bulimia nervosa and major depression: A study of common genetic and environmental factors. *Psychological Medicine, 22,* 617–622.

Weeks, D. E., Brzustowicz, L., Squires-Wheeler, E., Cornblatt, B., Lehner, T., Stefanovich, M., Bassett, A., Gilliam, T. C., Ott, J., & Erlenmeyer-Kimling, L. (1990). Report of a workshop on genetic linkage studies in schizophrenia. *Schizophrenic Bulletin, 16,* 673–686.

Weissman, M. M., Gammon, D., John, K., Merikangas, K. R., Warner, V., Prusoff, B. A., & Sholomskas, D. (1987). Children of depressed parents. Increased psychopathology and early onset of major depression. *Archives of General Psychiatry, 44,* 847–853.

Weissman, M. M., Gershon, E. S., Kidd, K. K., Prusoff, B. A., Leckman, J. F., Dibble, E., Hamovit, J., Thompson, W. D., Pauls, D. L., & Guroff, J. J. (1984). Psychiatric disorders in the relatives of probands with affective disorders: The Yale–NIMH collaborative family study. *Archives of General Psychiatry, 41,* 13–21.

Weissman, M. M., Prusoff, B. A., Gammon, G. D., Merikangas, K. R., Leckman, J. F., & Kidd, K. K. (1984). Psychopathology in the children (ages 6–18) of depressed and normal parents. *Journal of the American Academy of Child Psychiatry, 23,* 78–84.

Weissman, M. M., Wickramaratne, P., Adams, P. B., Lish, J. D., Horwath, E., Charney, D., Woods, S. W., Leeman, E., & Frosch, E. (1993). The relationship between panic disorder and major depression. A new family study. *Archives of General Psychiatry, 50,* 767–780.

Welner, Z., & Rice, J. (1988). School-aged children of depressed parents: A blind and controlled study. *Journal of Affective Disorders, 15,* 291–302.

Welner, Z., Welner, A., Stewart, M., Palkes, H., & Wish, E. (1977). A controlled study of siblings of hyperactive children. *Journal of Nervous and Mental Disease, 165,* 110–117.

Wender, P. H., Kety, S. S., Rosenthal, D., Schulsinger, F., Ortmann, J., & Lunde, I. (1986). Psychiatric disorders in the biological and adoptive families of adopted individuals with affective disorders. *Archives of General Psychiatry, 43,* 923–929.

Whitlock, F. A. (1982). *Symptomatic affective disorders.* New York: Academic Press.

Wilson, A. F., Elston, R. C., Siervogel, R. M., & Tran, L. D. (1988). Linkage of a gene regulating dopamine-beta-hydroxylase activity and the ABO blood group locus. *American Journal of Human Genetics, 42,* 160–166.

Winokur, G., & Coryell, W. (1991). Familial alcoholism in primary unipolar major depressive disorder. *American Journal of Psychiatry, 148,* 184–188.

Winokur, G., & Tanna, V. L. (1969). Possible role of X-linked dominant factor in manic depressive disease. *Diseases of the Nervous System, 30,* 89–94.

CHAPTER 6

Manic-Depressive Illness, Genes, and Creativity

KAY REDFIELD JAMISON

MANIC-DEPRESSIVE ILLNESS

The ethical issues surrounding any genetic illness are almost frighteningly complex. If the illness is common, treatable, displays itself in a wide range of behavioral, cognitive, and temperamental ways, and can confer advantage both to individuals and to their societies, then the ethical issues take on an entirely different level of complexity. This chapter, after giving a brief overview of manic-depressive illness, and its relationship to creativity, will discuss some of the potential problems, as well as benefits, underlying the search for the genes responsible for manic-depressive illness.

Manic-depressive, or bipolar, illness encompasses a wide range of mood disorders and temperaments. These vary in severity from cyclothymia—characterized by pronounced but not totally debilitating changes in mood, behavior, thinking, sleep, and energy levels—to extremely severe, life-threatening, and psychotic forms of the disease. Manic-depressive illness is closely related to major depressive, or unipolar, illness; in fact, the same criteria are used for the diagnosis of major depression as are used for the depressive phase of manic-depressive illness. These depressive symptoms include apathy, lethargy, hopelessness, sleep disturbance (sleeping

This chapter is excerpted from Jamison, K. R. (1993). *Touched with Fire: Manic-Depressive Illness and the Artistic Temperament.* New York: Free Press Macmillan.

KAY REDFIELD JAMISON • Department of Psychiatry, Johns Hopkins School of Medicine, Baltimore, Maryland 21218.
Genetics and Mental Illness: Evolving Issues for Research and Society, edited by Laura Lee Hall. Plenum Press, New York, 1996.

far too much or too little), slowed physical movement, slowed thinking, impaired memory and concentration, and loss of pleasure in normally pleasurable events. Additional diagnostic criteria include suicidal thinking, self-blame, inappropriate guilt, recurrent thoughts of death, a minimum duration of the depressive symptoms (2–4 weeks), and significant interference with the normal functioning of life. Unlike individuals with unipolar depression, those suffering from manic-depressive illness also experience episodes of mania or hypomania (mild mania). These episodes are characterized by symptoms that are, in many ways, the opposite of those seen in depression. Thus, during hypomania and mania, mood is generally elevated and expansive (or, not infrequently, paranoid and irritable), activity and energy levels are greatly increased, need for sleep is decreased, speech is often rapid, excitable, and intrusive, and thinking is rapid, moving quickly from topic to topic. Hypomanic or manic individuals usually have an inflated self esteem, as well as a certainty of conviction about the correctness and importance of their ideas. This grandiosity can contribute to poor judgment which, in turn, often results in chaotic patterns of personal and professional relationships. Other common features of hypomania and mania include spending excessive amounts of money, impulsive involvements in questionable endeavors, reckless driving, extreme impatience, intense and impulsive romantic or sexual liaisons, and volatility. In its extreme forms, mania is characterized by violent agitation, bizarre behavior, delusional thinking, and visual and auditory hallucinations. In its milder variants the increased energy, expansiveness, risk-taking, and fluency of thought associated with hypomania can result in highly productive periods. The range in severity of symptoms is reflected in the current psychiatric diagnostic system. Bipolar I disorder, what one thinks of as "classic" manic-depressive illness, refers to the most severe form of affective illness; individuals diagnosed as bipolar I must meet the full diagnostic criteria for both mania and major depressive illness. Bipolar II disorder, on the other hand, is defined as the presence or history of at least one major depressive episode, as well as the existence or history of less severe manic episodes (that is, hypomanias, which do not cause pronounced impairment in personal or professional functioning, are not psychotic in nature, and do not require hospitalization).

Cyclothymia, and related manic-depressive temperaments, are also an integral and important part of the manic-depressive spectrum, and the relationship of predisposing personalities and cyclothymia to the subsequent development of manic-depressive psychosis is a fundamental one. Cyclothymic temperament can be manifested in several ways: as predominantly depressive, manic, hypomanic, irritable, or cyclothymic. German psychiatrist Ernst Kretschmer (in Campbell, 1953) described the fluidity inherent to these manic-depressive temperaments:

Men of this kind have a soft temperament which can swing to great extremes. The path over which it swings is a wide one, namely between cheerfulness and unhappiness.... Not only is the hypomanic disposition well known to be a peculiarly labile one, which also has leanings in the depressive direction, but many of these cheerful natures have, when we get to know them better, a permanent melancholic element somewhere in the background of their being.... The hypomanic and melancholic halves of the cycloid temperament relieve one another, they form layers or patterns in individual cases, arranged in the most varied combinations.

Clearly, not all individuals who have cyclothymia go on to develop the full manic-depressive syndrome. But many do, and the temperamental similarities between those who meet all of the diagnostic criteria for mania or major depression (that is, "syndromal") and those who meet them only partially (that is, "subsyndromal" or cyclothymic) are compelling. British psychiatrists Dr. Eliot Slater and Sir Martin Roth have given a general description of the "constitutional cyclothymic," emphasizing the natural remissions, vague medical complaints, and seasonal patterns often intrinsic to the temperament. The alternating mood states—each lasting for days, weeks, or months at a time—are continuous in some individuals but subside, leaving periods of normality, in others. Slater and Roth (1969) also discuss the occurrence of the cyclothymic constitution in artists and writers:

Its existence in artists and writers has attracted some attention, especially as novelists like Bjørnsen and H. Hesse have given characteristic descriptions of the condition. Besides those whose swings of mood never intermit, there are others with more or less prolonged *intervals of normality*. In the hypomanic state the patient feels well, but the existence of such states accentuates his feeling of insufficiency and even illness in the depressive phases. At such times he will often seek the advice of his practitioner, complaining of such vague symptoms as headache, insomnia, lassitude, and indigestion.... In typical cases such alternative cycles will last a lifetime. In cyclothymic artists, musicians, and other creative workers the rhythm of the cycles can be read from the dates of the beginning and cessation of productive work. Some cyclothymic have a *seasonal rhythm* and have learned to adapt their lives and occupations so well to it that they do not need medical attention.

The distinction between full-blown manic-depressive illness and cyclothymic temperament is often an arbitrary one; indeed, almost all medical and scientific evidence argues for including cyclothymia as an integral part of the spectrum of manic-depressive illness. Such milder mood and energy swings often precede overt clinical illness by years (about one-third of those patients with definite manic-depressive illness, for example, report bipolar mood swings or hypomania predating the actual onset of their illness). These typically begin in adolescence or early adulthood and occur most often in the spring or autumn, on an annual or biennial basis. The symptoms, whose onset is usually unrelated to events in the individual's life, generally persist for 3 to 10 weeks, and are often characterized by changes in energy as well as mental discomfort. These subsyndromal mood swings, frequently debilitating, are as responsive to lithium treatment as full-blown manic-depressive illness is. In addition to the overlapping nature of symptoms in cyclothymia and manic-depressive illness, and the fact that cyclothymia responds to treatment with lithium, two further pieces of evidence support the relationship between the temperament and the illness. First, approximately 1 out of 3 patients with cyclothymia eventually develop full syndromal depression, hypomania, or mania; this is in marked contrast to a rate of less than 1 in 20 in control populations (Akiskal, Khani, & Scott-Strauss, 1979). Additionally, patients who have been diagnosed as cyclothymic have many more bipolar manic-depressive individuals in their family histories than would be expected by chance (Akiskal, Djenderendjian, Rosenthal, & Khani, 1977; DePue et al., 1981; Dunner, Russek, Russek, & Fieve, 1982). Particularly convincing are the data from studies of monozygotic (identical) twin pairs, which show that when one twin is diagnosed as manic-depressive, the other, if not actually manic-depressive, very frequently is cyclothymic (Bertelsen, Harvald, & Hauge, 1977).

Manic-depressive illness, often seasonal, is recurrent by nature; left untreated, individuals with this disease can expect to experience many, and generally worsening, episodes of depression and mania. It is important to note, however, that most individuals who have manic-depressive illness are normal most of the time; that is, they maintain their reason and their ability to function personally and professionally. Prior to the availability and widespread use of lithium, at least one person in five with manic-depressive illness committed suicide. The overwhelming majority of all adolescents and adults who commit suicide have been determined, through postportem investigations, to have suffered from either bipolar manic-depressive or unipolar depressive illness.

Manic-depressive illness is relatively common; approximately 1 person in 100 will suffer from the more severe form and at least that many again will experience milder variants, such as cyclothymia. One person in twenty will experience a major depressive illness. Men and women are equally likely to have manic-depressive illness, in contrast to major depressive illness, which is more than twice as likely to affect women. The average age of onset of manic-depressive illness (18 years) is considerably earlier than that of unipolar depression (27 years).

Highly effective treatments exist for both manic-depressive and major depressive illness. Lithium has radically altered the course and consequences of manic-depressive illness, allowing most patients to live reasonably normal lives. In recent years, anticonvulsant medications such as carbamazepine and valproate have provided important alternative treatments for patients unable to take, or unresponsive to, lithium. A wide variety of antidepressants has proven exceptionally powerful in the treatment of major depression. Psychotherapy, in conjunction with medication, is often essential to healing, as well as to the prevention of possible recurrences. Drug therapy, which is primary, frees most patients from the severe disruptions of manic and depressive episodes. Psychotherapy can help individuals come to terms with the repercussions of past episodes, take the medications that are necessary to prevent recurrence, and better understand and deal with the often devastating psychological implications and consequences of having manic-depressive illness.

MANIC-DEPRESSIVE ILLNESS AND CREATIVITY

Many highly creative and successful people have suffered extreme mood swings that are often serious enough to be described clinically as manic-depressive illness. Among 18th and 19th century British and American poets greatly impaired by their mood disorders were William Cowper, William Blake, Christopher Smart, John Clare, Lord Byron, Samuel Taylor Coleridge, Gerard Manley Hopkins, Herman Melville, Edgar Allan Poe, Dante Gabriel Rossetti, Percy Bysshe Shelley, and Alfred, Lord Tennyson. Twentieth century American poets John Berryman, Randall Jarrell, Robert Lowell, Theodore Roethke, Delmore Schwartz, and Anne Sexton all were hospitalized for mania, and Sylvia Plath for depression. Many of them also committed suicide.

Other manic-depressive or cyclothymic writers include Honoré de Balzac, Virginia Woolf, John Ruskin, F. Scott Fitzgerald, Charles Lamb, and Ernest Hemingway. Many composers also had significant mood disorders; among them were Orlandus Lassus, George Frideric Handel, Robert Schumann, Hector Berlioz, Gustav Mahler, Hugo Wolf, Gioacchino Rossini, Anton Bruckner, Peter Tchaikovsky, Alexsandr Scriabin, Edward Elgar, and Sergey Rachmaninoff.

The first scientific inquiries into the relationship between creativity and mood disorders were conducted in the 1970s. Using structured interviews, systematic diagnostic criteria, and matched control groups—a methodological advance over previous anecdotal research—Professor Nancy C. Andreasen at the University of Iowa (Andreasen, 1987) found an extraordinarily high rate of affective illness and alcoholism among creative writers. In her study, 24 of 30 writers (80%) had experienced at least one episode of affective illness; 43% reported periods of hypomania or mania as well. Consistent with a genetic basis, both creativity and affective disorders were also much more common in the relatives of writers than in the relatives of those in control groups.

I completed my own study of 47 British writers and visual artists while on sabbatical leave in England (Jamison, 1989). The artists and writers in my sample were chosen on the basis of acknowledged distinction in their fields. For example, all painters and sculptors were either Royal Academicians or associates of the Royal Academy, and all playwrights had won the New York Drama Critics Award and/or the Evening Standard Drama Award (London critics). Thirty-eight percent, a strikingly high percentage, had been treated for an affective illness. Three-fourths of those treated had been given antidepressant drugs or lithium, or had been hospitalized, or both.

Poets were the most likely to have required medication (33%); they were also the only ones (17%) who had required medical intervention for mania in the form of hospitalization, electroconvulsive therapy, or lithium. One-half of the poets had been treated with drugs or hospitalized for mood disorders.

Ruth Richards and her colleagues at Harvard have found that, compared with individuals who have no personal or family history of psychiatric disorders, manic-depressive and cyclothymic patients, as well as their not-ill relatives, show greater creativity (Richards *et al.*, 1988). University of Tennessee psychiatrist Hagop Akiskal and his colleagues interviewed 20 award-winning Parisian and other European writers, poets, painters, and sculptors; they found that recurrent cyclothymic or hypomanic tendencies occurred in nearly two-thirds of the sample and depressive episodes occurred in half (H. S. Akiskal, personal communication, 1988).

Biographical studies, as well as investigations conducted on living artists and writers, show a remarkable and consistent increase in rates of suicide, depression, and manic-depressive illness in highly creative groups—up to 18 times the rate of suicide in the general population, 8 to 10 times the rate of depression, and 10 to 20 times that of manic-depressive illness and its milder variants. The results from these studies are summarized in Figures 1 and 2.

How might a major mental disorder such as manic-depressive illness be linked to creativity? Profound changes in mood, thought, personality, and behavior can occur during all phases of the disorder. Probably most relevant to creativity are the mild manic states known as hypomania. In fact, formal diagnostic criteria for hypomania include elevated mood, increased self-esteem, high energy, decreased need for sleep, increased sexual desire, sharpened and unusually creative thinking, and increased productivity.

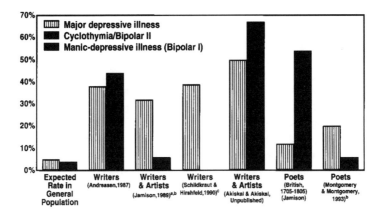

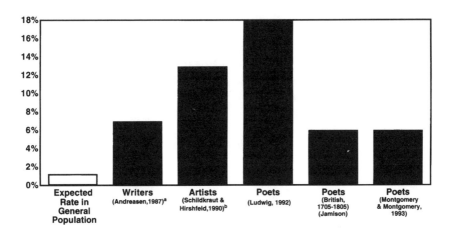

Figure 1.   Mood disorders in writers and artists. (Source: Jamison, *Touched with Fire*, 1993.)

Figure 2.   Suicide rates in writers and artists. (Source: Jamison, *Touched with Fire*, 1993.)

There is some evidence that expansiveness of thought and grandiosity of both mood and thought—common features of mild mania—result in an increased fluency and frequency of ideas that are highly conducive to creative achievement. The increase in speed of thoughts may range from a very mild quickening to complete psychotic incoherence. As the number of thoughts increases, unique ideas and associations may appear because of the qualitative changes in mental processing.

Manic-depressives illness, its associated temperaments, and creative accomplishment also have noncognitive features in common: the ability to function well on a few hours of sleep, to work at a high energy level, and to experience a great depth and variety of emotions.

THE GENETICS OF MANIC-DEPRESSIVE ILLNESS

Manic-depressive illness is a genetic disease, running strongly, not to say pervasively, in some families while absent in most. Robert Burton, as early as the 17th century, wrote unequivocally, "I need not therefore make any doubt of Melancholy, but that it is an hereditary disease," a view held by most medical observers long prior and long subsequent to his time. The inexorable passing on of madness from generation to generation is an ancient literary theme, as well as a traditional cultural and medical belief. Alfred, Lord Tennyson, who, as can be seen (Figure 3), had good reason to cast a brooding eye on his family's issue, spoke of a "taint of blood"; Lord Byron, of like vein but in a slightly different context, felt that "Some curse hangs over me and mine." And Edgar Allan Poe, of course, with a high sense of Gothic desolation and foreboding, described these family taints and curses in *The Fall of the House of Usher:*

During the whole of a dull, dark, and soundless day in the autumn of the year, when the clouds hung oppressively low in the heavens, I had been passing alone, on horseback, through a singularly dreary tract of country; and at length found myself, as the shades of the evening drew on, within view of the melancholy House of Usher. . . .

Its proprietor, Roderick Usher . . . spoke of acute bodily illness—of a mental disorder which oppressed him. . . .

I was at once struck with an incoherence—an inconsistency . . . an excessive nervous agitation. . . . His action was alternately vivacious and sullen. His voice varied rapidly from a tremulous indecision (when the animal spirits seemed utterly in abeyance) to that species of energetic concision . . . which may be observed in the lost drunkard, or the irreclaimable eater of opium, during the periods of his most intense excitement. . . .

It was, he said, a constitutional and a family evil, and one for which he despaired to find a remedy—

Modern medicine gives credence to these literary notions of familial madness; the genetic basis for manic-depressive illness is especially compelling, indeed almost incontrovertible.[1] Studies of identical and fraternal twins are a strong source of evidence for the heritability of manic-depressive illness. [Identical, or monozygotic, twins have the same genetic material whereas fraternal, or dizygotic, twins share only half of their genes (in this aspect, they are no different from other siblings); in contrast, both types of twins share a generally similar environment.] If one twin has manic-depressive illness, the other is far more likely (70 to 100%) to have it if the twins are identical than if they are fraternal (approximately 20%) (Bertelsen et al., 1977; Bertelsen, 1979; Mendlewicz, 1988; Gershon, 1990; Tsuang & Faraone, 1990). These concordance rates (the likelihood of a second twin being affected) for bipolar illness are much higher than those for unipolar depressive illness.[2] In an attempt to determine the relative importance of genetic as opposed to environmental influences, a few adoption studies have been carried out. A review of a total of 12 pairs of monozygotic twins who were reared apart from the time of infancy—and in which at least one of the twins had been diagnosed as having manic-depressive illness—found that 8 of the 12 pairs were concordant for the illness. This suggests a strong influence of genetic factors.

In family studies of mood disorders, researchers look for familial patterns in occurrence of mania, depression, and suicide. The many such studies that have been done are quite consistent in showing that manic-depressive

---

[1]Detailed reviews of this important but very complicated field of research can be found in Mendlewicz, J. (1988). Genetics of depression and mania. In A. Georgotas & R. Cancro (Eds.), *Depression and mania* (pp. 197–213), Amsterdam: Elsevier; Gershon, E. S. (1990). Genetics. In F. K. Goodwin & K. R. Jamison, *Manic-depressive illness* (pp. 373–401). London: Oxford University Press; Tsuang, M. T., & Faraone, S. V. (1990). *The genetics of mood disorders*. Baltimore: Johns Hopkins University Press; Winokur, G. (1991). *Mania and depression: A classification of syndrome and disease*. Baltimore: Johns Hopkins University Press.

[2]Tsuang, M. T., and Faraone, S. V. (1990). *The Genetics of Mood Disorders*. Baltimore: The Johns Hopkins University Press, p. 377. Drs. Larry Rifkin and Hugh Gurling of the Molecular Psychiatry Laboratory of University College and Middlesex School of Medicine in London have recently summarized the even stronger evidence for concordance in monozygotic twins: "Two series of twins selected on the basis of BP [bipolar] disorder probands have been the most thoroughly investigated over a particularly long time. These are the twins investigated by Bertelsen and those at the Maudsley Hospital. A recent reassessment of the Maudsley twins has now shown that the concordance for all subtypes of affective disorder in the co-twins is 100% [A. Reveley, 1990, personal communication]. Bertelsen [1988, personal communication] has also followed up his series of twins and if a diagnosis of suicide is counted as a case then the concordance amongst MZ twins is also 100%." Rifkin, L., & Gurling, H. (1991). Genetic aspects of affective disorders. In R. Horton & C. Katona (Eds.), *Biological aspects of affective disorders* (pp. 305–334; quoted on p. 313). New York: Academic Press.

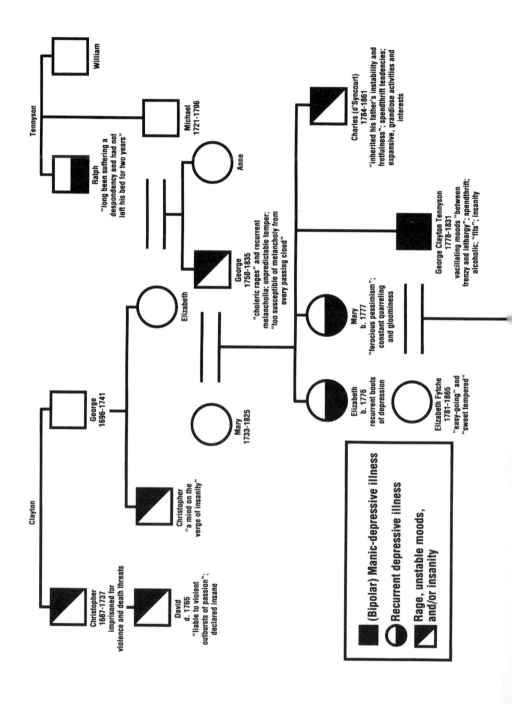

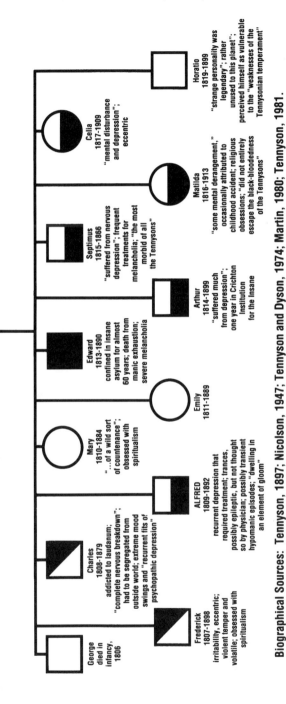

Biographical Sources: Tennyson, 1897; Nicolson, 1947; Tennyson and Dyson, 1974; Martin, 1980; Tennyson, 1981.

Figure 3.   Partial family history of Alfred, Lord Tennyson. (Source: Jamison, *Touched with Fire*, 1993.)

illness is indeed familial; the rate of manic-depressive and depressive illness in first-degree relatives of patients (that is, parents, siblings, and children) is far higher than the rate found in relatives of control groups.[3] Individuals who have manic-depressive illness are quite likely to have both bipolar and unipolar relatives. There is also some evidence that bipolar II illness (major depressive illness with a history of hypomania rather than mania) "breeds true"; that is, there is an increased risk of bipolar II illness among relatives of bipolar II patients (Gershon *et al.,* 1982; Coryell, Endicott, Reich, Andreasen, & Keller, 1984; Endicott *et al.,* 1985; De Paulo, Simpson, Gayle, & Folstein, 1990). Based on an extensive study of affectively ill patients, Dr. Elliot Gershon, chief of the Clinical Neurogenetics Branch of the National Institute of Mental Health, estimates that if one parent has manic-depressive illness and the other parent is unaffected, the risk of affective illness in the child (either depressive or manic-depressive illness) is 28%. If, however, both parents have affective illness and one of them is bipolar, it has been estimated that the risk of major depression or manic-depressive illness rises dramatically, to almost 75% (Gershon, 1990). There is a tendency for individuals with mood disorders to marry one another—"assortative mating"—and this has tremendous significance not only genetically but also psychologically for the children of such marriages.

A vigorous pursuit of the actual gene or genes responsible for manic-depressive illness is under way. In 1987 a group of investigators studying an Amish community in Pennsylvania reported a link between a dominant gene they thought conferred a predisposition to manic-depressive illness and chromosome 11 (Egeland *et al.,* 1987); at roughly the same time another team of researchers, studying an Israeli population, reported possible linkage on the X chromosome (Baron *et al.,* 1987; Mendlewicz *et al.,* 1987). Subsequent research has brought into question the validity of both the chromosome 11 and X chromosome findings (Hodgkins *et al.,* 1987; Kelsoe *et al.,* 1989; Berrettini *et al.,* 1990; Mendlewicz *et al.,* 1991), but few scientists in the field doubt that the gene—or, far more likely, the genes—for manic-

---

[3]The many family studies of manic-depressive illness are reviewed by Gershon in Goodwin and Jamison, *Manic-Depressive Illness.* Recent, well-controlled studies include Gershon, E. S., Hamovit, J. J., Guroff, E., Dibble, E., Leckman, J. F., Sceery, W., Targum, S. D., Nurnberger, J. I., Jr., Goldin, L. R., & Bunney, W. E., Jr. (1982). A family study of schizoaffective, bipolar I, bipolar II, unipolar, and normal control probands. *Archives of General Psychiatry, 39,* 1157–1167; Weissman, M. M., Gershon, E. S., Kidd, K. K., Prusoff, B. A., Leckman, J. F., Dibble, E., Hamovit, J., Thompson, W. D., Pauls, D. L., & Guroff, J. J. (1984). Psychiatric disorders in the relatives of probands with affective disorders: The Yale–National Institute of Mental Health collaborative study. *Archives of General Psychiatry, 41,* 13–21; Tsuang, M. T., Faraone, S. V., & Fleming, J. A. (1985). Familial transmission of major affective disorders: Is there evidence supporting the distinction between unipolar and bipolar disorders? *British Journal of Psychiatry, 146,* 268–271.

depressive illness will be found. Interestingly, a significant number of individuals who have the gene for manic-depressive illness, perhaps 20 or 30%, will never develop the disease. This so-called "incomplete penetrance," together with the tremendous range in the severity of the expression of the disease, raises central questions about the interactions between genetic predisposition, the physical and psychological environment (including stress, alcohol and other drugs, sleep loss, changing patterns of light, and psychological loss or trauma), and other protective or potentiating genes.

IMPLICATIONS

Occasionally an exhilarating and powerful creative force, more often a destructive one, manic-depressive illness gives a touch of fire to many of those who experience it. The melancholic side of manic-depressive illness is a source of intolerable suffering, torporous decay, and death; scarcely less damaging, mania in its extreme forms can be violently psychotic and life-threatening. Yet there is strong scientific and biographical evidence linking manic-depressive illness and its related temperaments to artistic imagination and expression. Biographies of eminent poets, artists, and composers attest to the strikingly high rate of mood disorders and suicide—as well as institutionalization in asylums and psychiatric hospitals—in these individuals, and recent psychiatric and psychological studies of living artists and writers have further documented the link. Manic-depressive illness, then, is a very strange disease—one that confers advantage but often kills and destroys as it does so. Not surprisingly, the clinical, ethical, and philosophical issues surrounding such a paradoxically advantageous and yet destructive illness are often difficult.

Very real issues of choice arise from the fact that manic-depressive illness is a genetic disease. These genetic issues are of considerably more long-term concern than the ones surrounding pharmacological treatments. Inevitably, given time and increasingly sophisticated research, the development of new drugs should make it possible to medicate individuals who have manic-depressive illness in such a way that the side effects are inconsequential and, it is to be hoped, in such a way that those aspects of temperament and cognition that are essential to the creative process will remain intact. The search for the gene or genes involved in manic-depressive illness raises far more difficult ethical problems, however; these issues become particularly complicated because manic-depressive illness can confer advantages on both the individual and society. Although unusual as a disease that brings with it certain advantages, it is by no means alone. Carriers of the sickle-cell trait, for example, appear to have relative immunity to certain types of malarial infections; in this context, Suzuki and Knudtson (1990) make the argument for a broad biological perspective when considering the notion of "defective genes":

> The story of sickle-cell anemia does underscore the striking capacity of a seemingly defective gene to simultaneously offer both advantages and disadvantages—depending on its quantities and surroundings. Moreover, there is growing evidence that natural selection often routinely maintains a balance of such mutant DNA sequences in populations of many species. The problem is that we are blind to that fragile balance except in rare instances, such as sickle-cell anemia, where geneticists have managed to unravel the intricacies of gene action in relation to hereditary disease.
>
> But how many other "defective" genes responsible for hereditary disorders might harbor some unseen evolutionary value? And, until we know enough about human genetics to begin to grasp their evolutionary roles, what price might we eventually pay if we overzealously try to "cure" these genetic abnormalities by ridding the human gene pool of these DNA sequences ... ?

Manic-depressive illness appears to convey advantage not only through its relationship to the artistic temperament and imagination, but also through its influence on many eminent scientists as well as business, religious, military, and political leaders (Goodwin & Jamison, 1990). Subtler effects that derive from its being a common illness with a wide range of temperamental and cognitive expression have yet to be assessed; indeed, few studies have examined the possible evolutionary reasons for the survival of *any* of the genes responsible for psychopathology, although some writers have suggested that schizophrenia, while devastating to those who suffer from it, might confer certain intellectual and temperamental advantages on first-degree relatives (Hammer & Zubin, 1968; Jarvik & Deckard, 1977; Sloman, Kanstantareas, & Dunham, 1979; Price & Sloman, 1984; Himmelhoch & Garfinkel, 1986). The complexities surrounding the search for the gene responsible for manic-depressive illness are enormous. It is highly unlikely, for example, that only one gene is involved and, even if an individual carries the gene (or genes), he or she may never become ill (likewise, he or she may or may not have the temperamental and cognitive characteristics associated with the illness). This suggests the likelihood of subtle, or not so subtle, interactions with the environment that might precipitate the first manic or depressive attack (for example, exposure to prolonged or significant changes in light, pronounced sleep reduction, drug or alcohol intake, childbirth) or the inheritance of other genes that might either trigger or protect against the disease. Physical and psychological factors also clearly play an important, although as yet unspecified role in the triggering and maintenance of, or protection against, the underlying genetic predisposition to manic-depressive illness. The complexity of locating the gene or genes underlying the inordinately broad range of temperamental, behavioral, and cognitive traits that constitute manic-depressive illness is beyond our current ability to imagine. Too, it is not unlikely that yet additional genetic, biochemical, and environmental factors may be at least in part responsible for both the illness and the cognitive and temperamental characteristics associated with artistic genius.

Several genetic issues are especially relevant to the diagnosis, treatment, and social policies surrounding manic-depressive illness; these include prenatal testing, abortion, forced sterilization, and gene therapy. Prenatal testing for manic-depressive illness and abortion based on a determination that a fetus is at risk for the disease may be choices that are available before the end of this century. The decision to abort a fetus obviously brings with it major ethical considerations, both for the parents involved and the society in which they live. Treatable common diseases, such as manic-depressive illness—ones that almost certainly confer societal and individual advantage and that vary greatly in the nature of their expression and their severity—are particularly problematic. Dr. Francis Collins, the medical geneticist at the University of Michigan who was instrumental in finding the genes for cystic fibrosis and neurofibromatosis, was asked in an interview (Collins, 1990) about prenatal testing for diseases that vary in severity or that first occur only later in life:

> This is where it gets muddy, and everyone is going to draw the line differently. Consider the situation with manic-depressive illness, a reasonably common disorder. It is clearly genetically influenced, though not in a simple way. Now, manic-depressive illness can be a terrible cross to bear. The swings into depression are awful, and the highs can be very destructive. Yet a substantial number of highly creative people have suffered from this disease. Suppose we find the gene responsible for manic depression. If every couple has a prenatal test to determine if a fetus is at risk for manic depression, and if every time the answer is yes that fetus is done away with, then we will have done something troubling, something with large consequences. Is this what we want to do?

Several related issues about prenatal testing have been raised, for example, the unclear boundaries between pathological conditions and normal traits, the important distinction between medically treatable and nontreatable genetic defects, the wide spectrum of severity of defects, and the variable ages of onset of the diseases in question. Larry Gostin, the director of the American Society of Law and Medicine, has addressed some of the difficult issues involved in genetic testing:

> Complex and often pernicious mythologies emerge from public ignorance of genetically-based diagnostic and prognostic tests. The common belief is that genetic technologies generated from scientific assessment are always accurate, highly predictive and capable of identifying an individual's or offspring's inevitable pre-destination of future disability. The facts are diametrically opposed to this common belief. The results of genetic-based diagnosis and prognosis are uncertain for many reasons.

> Predicting the nature, severity and course of disease based upon a genetic
> marker is an additional difficulty. For most genetic diseases the onset date,
> severity of symptoms, and efficacy of treatment and management are highly
> variable. Some people remain virtually symptom free, while others progress to
> seriously disabling illness. [Gostin, 1992]

Other scientists and ethicists have raised different concerns, including those of a more directly eugenic nature; for example, are there societal advantages to getting rid of certain genes altogether? On the other hand, might there be characteristics associated with a particular disease or trait that should be encouraged in the gene pool? It is of no little interest and irony that Francis Galton, a cousin of Charles Darwin and proponent of selective breeding in humans in order to obtain a "highly gifted race of man," was himself subject to "nervous breakdowns"; he was also appreciative of the "thin partitions" between greatness and psychopathology. Dr. Daniel Kevles, in his book *In the Name of Eugenics,* quotes Galton as saying that "men who leave their mark on the world are very often those who, being gifted and full of nervous power, are the same time haunted and driven by a dominant idea, and are therefore within a measurable distance of insanity." Involuntarily sterilization, a hallmark of the eugenics movement, and mandatory abortion seem highly unlikely options in this day and age, but many provinces in China still have government policies requiring individuals who have heritable mental illness (especially hereditary psychoses, which are of specific relevance to manic-depressive illness) to be sterilized; if pregnancy occurs, abortions are obligatory (Kristof, 1991). The historical precedent is chilling. Tens of thousands of mentally ill individuals, including many with manic-depressive illness, were sterilized or killed during the Third Reich, and many other thousands of psychiatric patients were sterilized earlier this century in the United States (Kevles, 1985). Ironically, one study carried out in Germany during the 1930s addressed the advisability of forced sterilization of individuals with manic-depressive illness. The author, who found that manic-depressive illness was greatly overrepresented in the professional and higher occupational classes, recommended against sterilization of these patients "especially if the patient does not have siblings who could transmit the positive aspects of the genetic heritage" (Luxenberger, 1993). During the 1940s, in a study undertaken by the Committee on Heredity and Eugenics, researchers at the McLean Hospital in Boston studied the pedigrees of several socially prominent American families. They came to a similar conclusion:

> Perhaps the words of Bumke need to be taken into account before we embark
> too whole-heartedly on any sterilization program, "If we could extinguish the
> sufferers from manic-depressive psychosis from the world, we would at the same

time deprive ourselves of an immeasurable amount of the accomplished and good, or color and warmth, of spirit and freshness." Finally, only dried up bureaucrats and schizophrenics would be left. Here I must say that I would rather accept into the bargain the diseased manic-depressive than to give up the healthy individuals of the same heredity cycle. [Myerson & Boyle, 1941]

Dr. John Robertson had written in like vein in his psychiatric study of Edgar Allan Poe 20 years earlier:

The qualities of the mind, as well as their morbid reactions, are too delicate ever to be understood or scientifically prearranged. For the world this is fortunate, however high an inheritance tax the victims of heredity must pay. Eradicate the nervous diathesis, suppress the hot blood that results from the overclose mating of neurotics, or from that unstable nervous organization due to alcoholic inheritance, or even from insanity and the various forms of parental degeneracy, and we would have a race of stoics—men without imagination, individuals incapable of enthusiasms, brains without personality, souls without genius. . . . Who could, or would, breed for a hump-backed Pope, or a clubfooted Byron, a scrofulous Keats, or a soul-obsessed Poe? Nature has done fairly well by us. [Robertson, 1923]

Debates about sterilization and forced abortion have been replaced, for the most part, by far more sophisticated debates about prenatal testing, voluntary abortions based on the results from such testing, and gene therapy. Many of the ethical problems remain very much the same, however.

Gene therapies comprise a variety of types of genetic manipulation, and all of them raise enormously complicated issues in their own right. The major ethical questions do not center primarily on the techniques designed to change the genetic code for only one individual (for example, inserting normal genes into a chromosome, removing defective genes, or using drugs that would treat genetic illnesses by "turning off" certain genes or "turning on" others). Even under those circumstances, however, one could argue about the advisability of changing genes that may be associated with subtle cognitive and temperamental characteristics vital to the well-being of society (including, for our discussion here, those related to the development of artistic imagination and expression). Certainly it is unclear what the alleviation of highly intense emotional experiences—including ecstatic or visionary states, psychosis, severe melancholia, or other types of mental suffering—might do to the ultimate nature of artistic expression as well as to the motivations underlying the production of works of art. The primary focus of ethical debate, however, is on those techniques that involve introducing genetically altered material into the reproductive cells (eggs and sperm), which could then be passed on to affect future generations as well. This, as Joel Davis points out, "violates the primary canon of human experimentation—the consent of the subject. The individual who agrees to have his or her germ cells changed can consent [depending on the age of the individual, of course]. *But that person's progeny are now committed to an experiment to which they did not consent"* [Davis, 1990]. Society, as well as the individual and his or her progeny, is bound to be deeply affected by decisions such as these.

Many of these ethical issues are being brought to the foreground by the Humane Genome Project, a vast 15-year program established by the U.S. government in 1990 with the goal of identifying the exact location and function of all of the genes in the human body. The potential benefits to health and basic science are largely obvious; without question, individuals who have genetic diseases—including those with manic-depressive illness—will gain immeasurably from the knowledge obtained about early identification and treatments, including the development of drugs that are based on an understanding of diseases at their molecular level. The mitigation of suffering and prevention of early death in those who have manic-depressive illness, or who are at risk for it, is a major public health priority. Although manic-depressive illness is much more common in writers and artists than in the general population, it would be irresponsible to romanticize an extremely painful, destructive, and lethal disease. Most people who suffer from manic-depressive and depressive illness are not unusually creative, and they reap few benefits from their experiences of mania and depression; even those who are highly creative usually seek relief from their suffering. Molecular biology research and the scientific advances ultimately provided by the mapping of the human genome have the potential to provide more specific, more effective, and less troubling treatments than now exist. Already, only 2 years after the Recombinant DNA Advisory Committee of the National Institutes of Health approved the first gene therapy trials in the United States, experimental treatment is being carried out in patients with cancer, diseases of the immune system, inherited high-cholesterol disorder, and other illnesses. Clinical trials have been proposed in several other countries and procedures viewed only a short time ago as radical and controversial are beginning to be used in medical research. The ethical ramifications of gene therapy and the Human Genome Project, however, are certainly far beyond our present capacity to comprehend. Because of the magnitude of potential social and ethical problems, 3 to 5% of the project's total budget (which is conservatively estimated at $3 billion) has been set aside for studies of the social, ethical, and legal implications of genetic research. This is an unprecedented commitment to ethical studies and will almost certainly ensure that troubling issues such as those we have been discussing will be examined at length and with subtlety. But they need to be raised and vigorously debated. While it is inconceivable that there will be any simple answer, awareness of the problem is a beginning. Dr.

James Watson, codiscoverer of the structure of DNA and the first director of the Human Genome Project, has made this point forcefully and repeatedly in his insistence on allocating massive resources to the study of ethical issues in genetic research:

> It would be nice to say that any of these answers are going to be simple. About all we can do is stimulate the discussion, and essentially lead the discussion instead of having it forced on us by people who say, "You don't know what you're doing." We have to be aware of the really terrible past of eugenics, where incomplete knowledge was used in a very cavalier and rather awful way, both here in the United States and in Germany. We have to reassure people that their own DNA is private and that no one else can get at it. We're going to have to pass laws to reassure them. [And] we don't want people rushing and passing laws without a lot of serious discussion first. [Watson, in Davis, 1990]

Fortunately, it seems more likely than not that the infinite varieties and complexities of life, with their infinite capacities for change, will be more rather than less recognized and appreciated as the genetic code begins to unwind:

> The real surprises, which set us back on our heels when they occur will always be the mutants. We have already had a few of these, sweeping across the field of human thought periodically, like comets. They have slightly different receptors for the information cascading in from other minds, and slightly different machinery for processing it, so that what comes out to rejoin the flow is novel, and filled with new sorts of meaning. Bach was able to do this, and what emerged in the current were primordia in music. In this sense, the Art of Fugue and the St. Matthew Passion were, for the evolving organism of human thought, feathered wings, apposing thumbs, new layers of frontal cortex. [Thomas, 1989]

Finally, there must be serious concerns about any attempt to reduce what is beautiful and original to a clinical syndrome, genetic flaw, or predictable temperament. It is frightening, and ultimately terribly boring, to think of anyone—certainly not only writers, artists, and musicians—in such a limited way. The fear that medicine and science will take away from the ineffability of it all, or detract from the mind's labyrinthine complexity, is as old as humanity's attempts to chart the movement of the stars. Even John Keats, who had studied to be a surgeon, felt that Newton's calculations would blanch the heavens of their glory. The natural sciences, he wrote, "will clip an Angel's wings,/Conquer all mysteries by rule and line,/Empty the haunted air, and gnomed mine—/Unweave a rainbow." What remains troubling is whether we have diminished the most extraordinary among us—our writers, artists, and composers—by discussing them in term of psychopathology or illnesses of mood. Do we—in our rush to diagnose, to heal, and perhaps even to alter their genes—compromise the respect we should feel for their differentness, independence, strength of mind, and individuality? Do we diminish artists if we conclude that they are far more likely than most people to suffer from recurrent attacks of mania and depression, experience volatility of temperament, lean toward the melancholic, and end their lives through suicide? I don't think so. Such statements seem to me to be fully warranted by what we now know; to deny them flies in the face of truth and risks unnecessary suffering, as well as not coming to terms with the important treatment and ethical issues that are raised by this complicated illness. American novelist Walker Percy, whose father and grandfather committed suicide and in whose family an unrelenting path of suicide, mania, and depression can be traced for at least 200 years, wrote:

> Death in the form of death genes shall not prevail over me, for death genes are one thing but it is something else to name the death genes and know them and stand over against them and dare them. I am different from my death genes and therefore not subject to them. My father had the same death genes but he feared them and did not name them and thought he could roar out old Route 66 and stay ahead of them or grab me and be pals or play Brahms and keep them, the death genes, happy, so he fell prey to them.
>
> Death in none of its guises shall prevail over me, because I know all the names of death. [Percy, 1981]

REFERENCES

Andreasen, N. C. (1987). Creativity and mental illness: Prevalence rates in writers and their first-degree relatives. *American Journal of Psychiatry, 144,* 1288–1292.

Akiskal, H. S., Djenderendjian, Rosenthal, R. H., & Khani, M. K. A. H., (1977). Cyclothymic disorder: Validating criteria for inclusion in the bipolar affective group. *American Journal of Psychiatry, 134,* 1227–1233.

Akiskal, H. S., Khani, M. K., & Scott-Strauss, A. (1979). Cyclothymic temperamental disorders. *Psychiatric Clinics of North America, 2,* 527–554.

Baron, M., Risch, N., Hamburger, R., Mandel, B., Kushner, S., Newman, M., Drumer, D., & Belmaker, R. H. (1987). Genetic linkage between X-chromosome markers and bipolar affective illness. *Nature, 326,* 289–292.

Berrettini, W. H., Golden, L. R., Gelernter, J., Gejman, P. V., Gershon, E. S., & Detera-Wadleigh, S. (1990). X-chromosome markers and manic-depressive illness: Rejection of linkage to Xq28 in nine bipolar pedigrees. *Archives of General Psychiatry, 47,* 366–373.

Bertelsen, A. (1979). A Danish twin study of manic-depressive disorders. In M. Schou & E. Strömgren (Eds.). *Prevention and treatment of affective disorders.* New York: Academic Press.

Bertelsen, A., Harvald, B., & Hauge, M. (1977). A Danish twin study of manic-depressive disorders. *British Journal of Psychiatry, 130,* 330–351.

Campbell, J. D. (1953). *Manic-depressive disease: Clinical and psychiatric significance.* Philadelphia: Lippincott.

Collins, F. (1990, September 17). Tracking down killer genes [interview with Dr. Collins], *Time,* p. 12.

Coryell, W., Endicott, J., Reich, T., Andreasen, N., & Keller, M. (1984). A family study of bipolar II disorder. *British Journal of Psychiatry, 145,* 49–54.

Davis, J. (1990). *Mapping the code: The Human Genome Project and the choices of modern science.* New York: Wiley.

De Paulo, J. R., Simpson, S. G., Gayle, J. O., & Folstein, S. (1990). Bipolar II disorder in six sisters. *Journal of Affective Disorders, 19,* 259–264.

De Pue, R. A., Slater, J. F., Wolfstetter-Kausch, H., Klein, D., Goplerud, E., & Farr, D. (1981). A behavioral paradigm for identifying persons at risk for bipolar depressive disorder: A conceptual framework and five validation studies. *Journal of Abnormal Psychology Monograph, 90,* 381–437.

Dunner, D. L., Russek, F. D., Russek, B., & Fieve, R. R. (1982). Classification of bipolar affective disorder subtypes. *Comprehensive Psychiatry, 23,* 186–189.

Egeland, J. A., Gerhard, D. S., Pauls, D. L., Sussex, J. N., Kidd, K. K., Allen, C. R., Hostetter, A. A., & Housman, D. E. (1987). Bipolar affective disorders linked to DNA markers on chromosome 11. *Nature, 325,* 783–787.

Endicott, J., Nee, J., Andreasen, N., Clayton, P., Keller, M., & Coryell, W. (1985). Bipolar II: Combine or keep separate? *Journal of Affective Disorders, 8,* 17–28.

Gershon, E. S. (1990). Genetics. In F. K. Goodwin & K. R. Jamison, *Manic-depressive illness.* London: Oxford University Press.

Gershon, E. S., Hamovit, J. J., Guroff, E., Dibble, E., Leckman, J. F., Sceery, W., Targum, S. D., Nurnberger, J. I., Jr., Goldin, L. R., & Bunney, W. E. (1982). A family study of schizoaffective, bipolar I, bipolar II, unipolar, and normal control probands. *Archives of General Psychiatry, 39,* 1157–1167.

Goodwin, F. K., & Jamison, K. R. *Manic-depressive illness. London: Oxford University Press.*

Gostin, L. (1992). Quoted in *Designing genetic information policy: The need for an independent policy review of the ethical, legal, and social implications of the Human Genome Project* (p. 24). Sixteenth report by the Committee on Government Operations. Washington, DC: U.S. Government Printing Office.

Hammer, M., & Zubin, J. (1968). Evolution, culture, and psychopathology. *Journal of General Psychology, 78,* 151–164.

Himmelhoch, J. M., & Garfinkel, M. E. (1986). Sources of lithium resistance in mixed mania. *Psychopharmacology Bulletin, 22,* 613–620.

Hodgkinson, S., Sherrington, R., Gurling, H., Marchbanks, R., Reeders, S., Mallet, J., McInnis, M., Petursson, H., & Brynjolfsson, J. (1987). Molecular genetic evidence for heterogeneity in manic depression. *Nature, 325,* 805–806.

Jamison, K. R. (1989). Mood disorders and patterns of creativity in British writers and artists. *Psychiatry, 52,* 125–134.

Jamison, K. R. (1993). *Touched with fire: Manic-depressive illness and the artistic temperment.* New York: Free Press Macmillan.

Jarvik, L. F., & Deckard, B. S. (1977). *Neuropsychobiology, 3,* 179–191.

Kelso, R., Jr., Ginns, E. I., Egeland, J. A., Gerhard, D. S., Goldstein, A. M., Bale, S. J., Pauls, D. J., Long, R. T., Kidd, K. K., Conte, G., Housman, D. E., & Paule, S. M. (1989). Reevaluation of the linkage relationship between chromosome 11p loci and the gene for bipolar affective disorder in the Old Order Amish. *Nature, 342,* 238–243.

Kevles, D. J. (1985). *In the name of eugenics: Genetics and the uses of human heredity.* New York: Knopf.

Kristof, N. D. (1991, August 15). Parts of China forcibly sterilizing the retarded who wish to marry. *New York Times,* pp. A1, A8.

Ludwig, A. M. (1992). Creative achievement and psychopathology: Comparisons among professions. *American Journal of Psychotherapy, 46,* 330–356.

Luxenberger, H. (1933). Berufsglied und soziale Schichtung in den Familien erblich Geisteskranker. *Eugenik, 3,* 34–40.

Martin, R. B. (1980). *Tennyson: The unquiet heart.* Oxford: Clarendon Press.

Mendlewicz, J. (1988). Genetics of depression and mania. In A. Georgotas & R. Cancro (Eds.), *Depression and Mania* (pp. 197–213). Amsterdam: Elsevier.

Mendlewicz, J., Leboyer, M., De Bruyn, A., Malafosse, A., Sevy, S., Hirsch, D., van Broeckhovem, C., & Mallet, J. (1991). Absence of linkage between chromosome 11p15 markers and manic-depressive illness in a Belgian pedigree. *American Journal of Psychiatry, 148,* 1683–1687.

Mendlewicz, J., Simon, P., Sevy, S., Charon, F., Brocas, H., Legros, S., & Vassart, G. (1987). Polymorphic DNA marker on X chromosome and manic depression. *Lancet, 1,* 1230–1232.

Myerson, A., & Boyle, R. D. (1941). The incidence of manic-depressive psychosis in certain socially important families. *American Journal of Psychiatry, 98,* 11–21.

Nicolson, H. (1947). *Tennyson's two brothers: The Leslie Stephen Lecture 1947.* London: Cambridge University Press.

Percy, W. (1981). *The second coming* (p. 314). New York: Washington Square Press/ Pocket Books.

Poe, E. A. (1839). *The fall of the house of Usher and other writings* (pp. 138–145). Reprint, New York: Penguin Books, 1986.

Price, J. S., & Sloman, L. (1984). The evolutionary model of psychiatric disorder. *Archives of General Psychiatry, 41,* 211.

Richards, R. L., Kinney, D. K., Lunde, I., Benet, M., & Merzel, A. P. (1988). Creativity in manic-depressives, cyclothymes, their normal relatives, and control subjects. *Journal of Abnormal Psychology, 97,* 281–288.

Robertson, J. W. (1923). *Edgar A. Poe: A psychopathic study,* (p. 145). New York: Putnam.

Schildkraut, J. J., Hirshfeld, A. J., & Murphy, J. (1994). Mind and mood in modern art II: Depressive disorders, spirituality and early deaths in the abstract expressionist artists of the New York School. *American Journal of Psychiatry, 151,* 482–488.

Slater, E., & Roth, M. (1969). *Clinical psychiatry* (3rd ed., pp. 206–207). Baltimore: Williams & Wilkins.

Sloman, L., Konstantareas, M., & Dunham, D. W. (1979). The adaptive role of maladaptive neurosis. *Biological Psychiatry, 14,* 961–972.

Suzuki, D., & Knudtson, P. (1990). *Genetics: The clash between the new genetics and human life* (pp. 183–184). Cambridge: Harvard University Press.

Tennyson, C., & Dyson, H. (1974). *The Tennysons: Background to genius.* London: Macmillan.

Tennyson, H. (1897). *Alfred Lord Tennyson: A memoir.* London: Macmillan.

Tennyson, H. (Ed.) (1981). *Studies in Tennyson.* London: Macmillan.

Thomas, L. (1989). Notes of a biology watcher: To err is human. In B. Dixon (Ed.), *From creation to chaos: Classic writings in science* (pp. 199–201). Oxford: Basil Blackwell.

Tsuang, M. T., & Faraone, S. V. (1990). *The genetics of mood disorders.* Baltimore: Johns Hopkins University Press.

Watson, J. D., quoted in Davis, J. (1990). *Mapping the code: The Human Genome Project and the choices of modern science* (p. 262). New York: Wiley.

CHAPTER 7

A Hunger for Knowledge and Respect

MARY ANN BEALL

In January, 1993, the congressional Office of Technology Assessment held the first major meeting on genetics and mental illness to invite to the table, on an equal footing with world-class researchers, those most profoundly affected by the topic at hand: people with severe mental illness and our families. This inclusiveness challenges discriminatory assumptions, prejudices, and oversimplification of complex etiologies which have dogged the quest to eradicate major mental illness, and still dog us, who have no choice but to live in the belly of that beast.

Research and new knowledge open doors on recovery for people like me. New genetic findings gave me critical insight into my disorder which was essential for me to understand and accept the first effective treatment I ever experienced. It put my mental illness in a comprehensible context, my behaviors and thost of my family became understandable, fully human. After half a century of grim suffering, my life became worth fighting for once again.

This chapter will touch on four considerations: the disconnect between research and public mental health systems where most people with severe

MARY ANN BEALL • Virginia Alliance for the Mentally Ill, Richmond, Virginia 23215.

Genetics and Mental Illness: Evolving Issues for Research and Society, edited by Laura Lee Hall. Plenum Press, New York, 1996.

psychiatric disabilities are treated; the issues most important to consumers, in their own words; the dysfunctional public system and how and in what context genetic services might be provided to really help consumers; and the quintessential importance of genetic information in my recovery.

Long after the workshop I was troubled by aching questions. If those searching for answers don't know us, or how we really live, or what we think and feel, how likely is what they find, particularly if it's of great importance, to be effectively targeted to reach us? What happens to us while we wait?

INVISIBLE PEOPLE: PEOPLE WITH MENTAL ILLNESS

I was nervous, exhilarated to be at the table that gray morning at OTA. Yet as the meeting unfolded I was shocked by how wide the gap was between the insular academic world of the researcher and the daily struggle of families and consumers to obtain effective, humane treatment. The unwitting ignorance of so many in that room about who consumers are and what we experience was vastly disconcerting.

I know that we, particularly the most seriously affected, live extraordinarily isolated lives, denied the most commonly shared adult experiences: a home, meaningful work, marriage, advanced education, skills training, friends, children, even pets (Beall, 1993a). We live in segregated contexts even outside state hospitals. We live with our parents long after it's socially appropriate or in residential programs in the community, but still have little contact with those who live in the "normal" world around us.

Isolation functions to reinforce simplistic notions of who we are, what we need, and what we experience (Beall, 1993a; Campbell & Schraiber, 1989; Marsh, 1994; Peet, 1993). Clinical staff and researchers often see just fragments of our lives, and assume they know and understand far more than they actually do. They've been known to mistake an embellishment for a major motif, a part of our lives for the whole (Beall, 1993a; Bevilacqua, 1992; Campbell, Ralph, & Glover, 1994; Trochim, Dumont, & Campbell, 1993).

What compounds misunderstanding is an assumption that one consumer is much like the next. It's impossible to generalize about us. Each of us is unique. Mental illness is not a static disability. Our symptoms change over time and we experience our disorders in extremely diverse ways. A consumer with my diagnosis can have very different symptoms, and gravely disabling side effects from the identical dose of medication that currently works extremely well, with no side effects for me (Campbell & Frey, 1993).

We have inordinately wide ranges of ability and disability. These disorders emerge in adolescence and young adulthood, so we come with widely different educational backgrounds, ranging from fragments of elementary education to multiple graduate degrees. Consumers and families find it no great surprise that data from genetic research imply heterogeneity.

LIFTING THE CLOAK OF SILENCE: MAKING THE INVISIBLE, VISIBLE

The real lives of people with severe psychiatric disabilities are starkly outlined in the results of a survey conducted by the Virginia Mental Health Consumers Association. In November, 1992, VMHCA sent 1700 questionnaires to people with major mental illness served by the Virginia Department of Mental Health, Mental Retardation and Substance Abuse Services (Beall, 1993a). In 10 days, over 600 completed surveys were back at the Association offices. The quality of the returns and their sheer numbers stunned us. We'd not included stamped or addressed return envelopes with the survey and most consumers live in such dire poverty that the cost of a stamp can be prohibitive (Beall, 1993a,b).

Reading the individual forms was humbling and emotionally wrenching. The other readers and I found ourselves constantly in tears of anguished identification and remembrance. Along with grief and pain came the incredible realization, "We're not alone." There were many others whose life experiences and feelings were identical to our own—our isolation was shattered.

> If we could get real help before we are desperate and too sick, we would not have to be in the hospital so often.
>
> I wish staff could view us as human and not discourage friendship or act so ashamed of us.
>
> Since I have been sick I have lived in poverty and fear.
>
> I hope someone in Richmond has a conscience.
>
> Consumers need encouragement and much more information about our disorders, medications, treatment, so we can make real choices that impact our treatment.
>
> More accurate earlier diagnosis, [to] reduce hospitalizations and inappropriate treatments.
>
> Qualified staff educated about mental illnesses.
>
> I need to continue looking for the right combination of medications to manage my illness. Most doctors here are, well, less than 'cutting edge'. Frankly, they are terrible.
>
> I am not an animal! Stop punishing me. Try to help me.
>
> I need help in understanding how medications are supposed to work, and when to ask for help. [Many consumers said this.]
>
> We need better hospital programs that will really help us manage our mental illnesses better. Real education that will help us do better in the community and in our real lives.

We want what all human beings want: homes, friends, love, work, and
even more basic things.

> Food. I go hungry too much.
>
> I'm so alone since I got sick.
>
> I am really afraid of the place I have to live. They do drugs all over here.

In addition to documenting lives of crushing poverty and deprivation,
what leapt off those survey response sheets was our sheer hunger for
knowledge, for respect (Beall, 1993a,b).

We're unique individuals and don't fit under any single rubric. What
people with severe psychiatric disabilities have in common is that we suffer stigma, discrimination, abject poverty, social isolation, and misunderstanding. Above all else we need effective medical treatment, to have our
needs met in ways that respect our dignity as human beings. We want to
access effective services and treatments able to help us recover our lives.
We yearn for knowledge and the benison of healing.

As long as I thought my suffering was unique to me, the true magnitude
of the catastrophic state in which people like me existed was invisible even
to me. I suffered in silent shame, alone. When I was handed confirmation
of our grim common reality, I began to question basic assumptions about
people like me and about the system that "treats" us.

THE CONSEQUENCES OF INVISIBILITY

When one of the best-known researchers at the OTA workshop mentioned in passing that "patients actually don't want genetic counseling"
(Gershon, 1993), I found myself taking a deep breath. This flies in the face
of consumer concerns plainly stated in the VMHCA Survey. People with
mental illness want to know everything: the simple, the complex, the sure,
the unsure.

We burn with hope that someday we'll be able to say with Nancy
Andreasen, author of *The Broken Brain,* "My life has always been shaped
by the Baconian dictum that 'knowledge is power.' If I knew what was
happening and what was going to happen, I could be confident and un-
afraid" (Andreasen, 1984; Beall, 1993a).

Lack of access to and knowledge about newer, more effective treatments for mental illness plus the generally poor quality of public psycho-
pharmacologic services and lack of primary medical care have as much
negative impact on consumer quality of life as major mental illness itself
(Beall, 1993a; Flynn, 1993).

Some of the most punishing things consumers suffer are iatrogenic,
inflicted on us by the very system founded to help us, to care for us. Most

of what historically determined the structure of public mental health service systems has in the light of current scientific research turned out to be not only wrongheaded but also false (Marsh, 1994; Peavey, 1994; Shamoo & Irving, 1993).

Outrage at the helpless suffering of people with severe mental illness moved those who love us to found our rapidly growing national grass roots movement, 140,000 strong. The National Alliance for the Mentally Ill dedicates its existence to scientific research, to seeking effective treatments, to eradicating mental illness, to ending prejudice and discrimination (Flynn, 1993). For 15 years NAMI members, families and consumers, have worked tirelessly in support of scientific research to uncover the root causes of and discover the cures for these catastrophic brain disorders, as well as for service system reform, and much needed changes in professional curricula and training (Flynn, 1993).

NAMI has greatly expanded the funding base for research, which has confirmed that the severe mental illnesses, although of complex etiology, are disorders of the brain.

As the revolution in molecular genetic technology focuses on identifying genetic contributions to severe psychiatric disabilities, and as new data identify the biological substrate and actual biological mechanisms that cause severe and persistent mental illness, the issue of whether mental illnesses are "real physical illness" has finally been put to rest (Gottesman, 1991).

The Human Genome Project, the Decade of the Brain, the discovery of better and more effective treatments are drivers in moving public attitudes about mental illness. Science has had great power to reduce the scapegoating of families and consumers and public attitudes are changing for the better (Clements, 1993; Flynn, 1993; Folstein, 1993).

THE POLITICS OF INVISIBILITY: A DYSFUNCTIONAL SERVICE SYSTEM

The overwhelming reality that survey respondents described is a public mental health treatment system that is disjointed, out of touch, and too often pathogenic. The new knowledge base about the nature of major mental illness revealed in the past 10 to 15 years hasn't impacted treatment practices in most public systems that consumers and families use daily (Beall, 1993a; Biesecker, 1993; Flynn, 1993; Trochim *et al.*, 1993).

Never before in human history has there been such a wealth of information about or such a huge and effective armamentarium available to overcome the effects of severe mental illness. Severely disabled people, who in the past would have had no choice but to suffer the scourge of major mental illnesses, should be the beneficiaries of the new knowledge and should be experiencing recovery and returning to productive lives. Recovery should be as common as weeds. But it isn't.

In Richmond, Virginia, hundreds of consumers have been screened for Clozaril over the past few years, but only three are currently accessing it. It's like routinely using leeches rather than operating on people in need of heart bypass surgery.

The transfer of new knowledge and technology with such dramatic potential to relieve so much suffering for those served by public mental health systems is proceeding at a glacial pace. There is an abyss between academic centers of excellence where new discoveries are being made, and the public treatment systems which should be rushing to embrace new knowledge and better treatments but which, incomprehensibly, are not.

The discoveries of neurobiological research and molecular genetics most often reach consumers only via the media (Green, 1994).

As Robert D. Coursey of the Psychology Department at the University of Maryland observes, "As teachers, service providers, and researchers concerned with serious mental illness, we are continually challenged to re-evaluate much of what we have traditionally been taught to think and do. Indeed, many researchers and practitioners who work with people who have serious mental illness are laboring under old viewpoints that are unproductive and that misrepresent the phenomena that we are attempting to understand and treat" (Marsh, 1994).

Other currents are sweeping through society. These are uncertain times, and our nation has yet to resolve the crisis in funding all medical care. Even so, we live in a time of miracles. My recovery and the recovery of others are testament to that, but there is a real chance society may choose not to foot the bill for new effective treatments to be made available to those who need and would benefit from them most.

The private treatment system over the past decade has moved to control costs, by limiting the definition and number of services covered and via managed care. There has been significant decrease in private insurance coverage for people with major mental illness, and the transfer of the most seriously ill to public systems of care continues apace (Rodgers, Wells, Merideth, & Sturm, 1993).

People who aren't seriously disabled or are able to work full time, or with private resources, are the only ones who can avoid public system care. De facto segregation of the two systems is stratified by diagnosis and severity of disability (Beall, 1993b; Flynn, 1993).

Moves to cut costs by insurers have resulted in severely mentally ill people receiving less than adequate care (Rodgers *et al.*, 1993). As time passes we learn of more consumers denied appropriate treatment who've lost their lives, apparently as a result.

Tragically, it is not clear that the currently fragmented, chaotic public treatment systems, if they were reorganized and required to offer quality treatment of proven scientific efficacy, would cost more than they currently do. This is certainly not the case in human costs and may not be so for truly effective, coordinated care.

The difficulty is not just technology and knowledge transfer, i.e., straightforward systems reform, it is complicated by partisan politics. Public treatment systems are at the beck and call of politicians who appoint state commissioners of mental health. Ideology and politics thus drive systems that should be driven by best medical practices, excellence of care, rehabilitation, normalization, and, most of all, recovery.

To put this in context, the new commissioner of my state's mental health system earnestly explained to me soon after he was appointed that the major new initiative he wanted to launch was to prevent major psychiatric disabilities such as schizophrenia by making more marriage counseling available to young couples.

State mental health systems have proved extraordinarily hard to reform and to make accountable for the efficacy of care they provide. Resistance to collecting data that would reveal whether the services they provide actually result in positive outcomes for people with severe mental illness is ubiquitous (Campbell & Frey, 1993; Campbell et al., 1994).

There are immense pressures in public systems which silence those of us who receive services and keep us from asking questions or speaking openly about our experiences. If we speak out, we risk swift retaliation (Beall, 1993a; Tanzman, 1990). The public system is the court of last resort, however inappropriate, out of date, or actually harmful. If we don't do as we're told, we risk being actively pushed out on the streets and losing all hope of any help.

In the late 1980s a few academic researchers began to poll consumers on our needs and preferences and it became clear that we are silenced by fear. We don't ever tell people who run the treatment system what we think about their pervasive disdain for us or how often the systems catastrophically fail us (Beall, 1993a; Campbell & Schraiber, 1989; Tanzman, 1990).

Researchers had to exert extraordinary effort to ensure that consumers felt safe enough to share the truth of their lives and what they needed to recover and maintain stable well-being in the community. The Center for Community Change in Vermont and the Well Being Project in California broke ground in this regard. Both efforts used consumers extensively in the construction of survey instruments as well as for interviewers (Campbell & Schraiber, 1989; Tanzman, 1990).

When we're safe from retaliation, we tell the truth, and it's clear we've thought long and hard about how to make the public treatment system humane and successful. We can be characterized as terribly frustrated collaborators (Tanzman, 1990). No group of people want this public system to work really well more than do consumers and our families.

GENETIC COUNSELING: OPENING THE DOOR TO ACCEPTANCE

Any move to provide genetic information to people with psychiatric disabilities and their family members must be reality tested. To be effective, genetic services must take into account the dire straits consumers exist in, their hunger for information, and the lamentable state of public treatment systems.

The paramount issue to factor into genetic counseling is knowledge of and respect for the complex and difficult process of personally accepting one's mental illness, and the importance of setting the stage for our positive active involvement in treatment. Acceptance is a process, not a simple single event.

There are other monkey wrenches in the works which must be factored in, such as the powerful prohibitions against acknowledging, no less accommodating, the sexual needs of adults with major mental illness. Sex and parenthood are absolute taboos. Equally powerful is a long history of abuse, and the discriminatory potential of genetic information.

PARTNERS IN HEALING

In an ideal treatment system, counseling an individual on the risks of inheriting major mental illnesses should be triggered by the consumer, or by the family (Flynn, 1993; Pardes, 1993; Sapers, 1994; Tsuang, 1993).

However, in this very imperfect world there are such major discontinuities in public treatment systems that this could prove a very poor strategy. The people who work directly with us are mostly aides or those with little professional training. Also the process of getting an accurate diagnosis is often a protracted, torturous process. A consumer from Petersburg, Virginia, told it like it is: "The medical doctors in state hospitals are often out of date and uninformed. Too many of us waste years struggling not only with our disabilities but with treatments bound to fail, because it takes so very long to get accurately diagnosed. In my case it took twenty years to sort through about as many false diagnoses. It's an outrage" (Beall, 1993a,b).

In the public treatment system in Virginia, there is little contact between consumers and their families and physicians or others who might be qualified or credentialed to do genetic counseling. Consumers in the community are lucky if we see a psychiatrist 10 minutes every 3 months. That's not enough time to do adequate psychopharmacological care, no less anything else (Beall, 1993a).

Yet I believe genetic services are crucial, both in helping us to understand our disorders and in helping us constructively accept our disabilities so we can begin the process of recovery. How information is shared can set the stage so that it is possible for us to invest in our treatment as full partners. For that to happen, traditional power relationships must change, from "doing to," or "doing for," to "doing with." Consumers must be able to rebuild trust with professionals in order to be active partners in treatment (Beall, 1993b; Bevilacqua, 1992).

As Drs. Diamond and Factor (1994) observe in an editorial in *Hospital and Community Psychiatry,* titled "Treatment Resistant Patients or a Treatment Resistant System?," "As we continue to work with patients, we are struck by how the use of certain language can restrict our thinking and interfere with our ability to provide effective treatment." They point out that "the problem is not that . . . patients refuse treatment, but rather that they do not want to 'buy' the treatment we want to 'sell'. Actually, many of them later accept medication after they have developed a trusting relationship with us and learn we will help them with their agendas before imposing our own" (Diamond & Factor, 1994).

Too many of the psychiatrically disabled living on the streets are people who have been abandoned or actively rejected by public treatment systems. Consumers and families know, the more socially impaired, the less likely you are to be served (Beall, 1993a). Once a consumer is tagged as "uncooperative" or "treatment resistant," it can become impossible for them to access any care. People who experience multiple rejections by the treatment system often cease to be able to participate in any constructive way in self-care (Beall, 1993a; Trochim *et al.,* 1993).

Recent polls of consumers who attend affective disorders support and self-help groups show that 88 to 92% indicated that they would have genetic testing as soon as it became available (Sapers, 1994).

This confirms earlier surveys of people at risk for Huntington's chorea. Even at this time, with no effective treatment available, fully 80% wanted testing and wanted no information withheld from them. They felt the decision to withhold should *not* be left to medical professionals (Sapers, 1994).

There is no question we yearn for knowledge, to know the risks and the uncertainties, for how else can we recover our lives (Beall, 1993b)? Yet, the issues remain of who, when, where and how?

Far too little attention has been paid on the part of treatment professionals and researchers to the early stages of these disorders. The multiple processes of understanding and accepting that one or one's family member has a major mental illness are not well understood.

We do know, above all else, that acceptance is a complex, time-consuming process, on which our very lives depend. Our extremely varied levels of ability and disability dictate that this must be an individualized process.

We know that acceptance, as it has played out in the past, has been a devastating time, which some of us don't survive, or survive so impaired, in such denial, we can't take any meaningful role in our continuing treatment (Beall, 1993a; Coursey, Farrell, & Zahniser, 1991; Flynn, 1993; Weiden, 1994).

We go through stages of acceptance, and denial, some of which parallel Kubler-Ross's stages in accepting death, and dying. Who I believed I am, who I believed I would be, will never happen. In despair and too often alone we die to ourselves. We die to our hopes. We die to our family's hopes yet we continue to breathe, to be alive. Somehow we must continue to find life in the ruin of all our hopes (Beall, 1993b).

Researchers and professionals need to learn from those of us with severe psychiatric disabilities who are recovering good quality of life, so they can begin to identify the critical factors in positive acceptance and recovery, and, in turn, replicated the latter for others (Beall, 1993a; Spaniol & Kechler, 1994).

PRIMAL TABOOS: SEXUALITY AND PARENTHOOD

At a number of points during formal presentations at OTA the presumption went unchallenged that for people with serious psychiatric disabilities the result of genetic counseling would be to forgo childbearing or marriage (Flynn, 1993; Folstein 1993; Gershon, 1993).

Reproduction and sexuality have always proved the skunk at the garden party, as they have for all people with profound disability. Most residential programs serving consumers are sex segregated, and the fastest way to end up on the streets is to be an obviously sexually active adult.

When we do have children, they're often taken from us, not necessarily because of concrete evidence that we are inadequate parents but because departments of welfare still operate on the stigmatic assumption that to have a diagnosis of major mental illness is to be incompetent, incapable of loving, or unable to parent responsibly. Accusations of parental unfitness are staple fodder in contested divorce cases and don't have much to do with psychiatric disability. The issue for us, as it is for all parents with major disabling conditions, is the quality and availability of assistance and individualized support.

It is almost impossible to describe the coercion to relinquish her child faced by a pregnant woman with a major psychiatric disorder in many public programs.

For people with major mental illness this kind of coercion wears so many masks: from very subtly distorted assumptions applied to us, to our being helplessly subject to the inhuman and inhumane. I don't believe there are enough tears in this universe to fill these wells of grief. "I am so desperate to see my children. D.S.S. has taken them because I have depression. I may have a mental illness, but I would never, never hurt them. I love them so much" (Beall, 1993a).

The unspoken disregard for our sexual needs and our adulthood undergirds what many of us feel is the most appalling example of how our sexuality is discounted and ignored and how we are negatively labeled and treated in ways that have far-reaching and sometimes fatal consequences. The impact on young male consumers' willingness to accept a diagnosis that may leave them no choice but to risk the most commonly unacknowledged side effect of first-generation neuroleptics is a prime example of how casually we are disregarded and devalued.

The side effect that professionals rarely publicly acknowledge or address is complete sexual dysfunction. Just how many adolescents or young men would willingly accept a label that consigns them to that? How long would medication to treat any other common disorder stay on the market with that downside? It amazes me that professionals continue to blame "medication noncompliance" on "treatment-resistant patients" never considering how long they would tolerate this particular side effect themselves.

Keep in mind, half of all people prescribed nonpsychiatric prescriptions don't finish the pills in the bottle, even if the medications are effective and have no significant side effects.

CAUTION: GENETIC INFORMATION INSIDE

Historically, genetics has proved a wickedly double-edged tool in the search for a way to eradicate severe psychiatric disabilities. Yet paradoxically, molecular genetics possesses unusual power to demystify major mental illnesses and to refute stigma. Widespread publicity about genetic contributions to affective disorders has proved key to reducing the intensity of stigma associated with depressive and manic-depressive disorders (Clements, 1993; Cook-Deegan, 1993; Flynn, 1993).

Nonetheless, uneasiness and downright confusion pervade large sectors of our society, fueled by fears that the technological revolution in molecular genetics will be used, at this end of this century, either to block access to care, or to limit availability to a full range of medical services based on some calculation of genetic risk. There remain suspicions that genetics might find itself used to justify some form of institutionalized discrimination, as it did early in this century, under the rubric of eugenics (Cook-Deegan, 1993; Flynn, 1993).

Ironically, eugenics originated in the benign hope of reducing human suffering by encouraging the birth of healthy children. The very word comes from *eu* and *genes,* which mean "wellborn" in ancient Greek. Eugenics became a popular social and political movement shored up by simplistic notions of race and genetic inheritance welded to an intense faith in the power of prevention and mental hygiene current in the early 1900s.

From the conjoining of these ideologies, it was but a small side step into serious consideration of improving the quality of human bloodlines and races by superior genetic selection, as well as the duty to discourage the reproduction of inferior peoples.

There was just enough science in the admixture to lend credibility, even respectability, to those advocating the policies and practice of eugenics. So the door edged upon on one of the most shameful chapters in human history. We consumers will never forget that it was mentally disabled people just like us who led that terrible parade to the death camps in the 1930s.

The shadow cast by the politics of eugenics swept wide in this country where discrimination on the basis of race has always defined such a catalysmic divide.

Eugenic ideology became and remains widely enshrined in state codes. Even as we met in 1992 at OTA, some states still had compulsory sterilization laws on their books (Beall, 1993b).

As little as 20 years ago it took litigation, with large punitive damages, to end routine forced sterilization of people with mental illness in public mental hospitals in my home state. Such sterilization was performed on people whose consent was never sought, and most of whom were never informed of what had been done to them. The settlement mandated the state to tell consumers the truth about what had been done to them. Several personal friends were among those notified (Beall, 1993b).

Unfortunately, prejudice and some of the oldest stigmatic canards retain surprising currency in the popular culture of the conservative right. Year after year, disquieting discriminatory practices find their way into state codes. We can't afford to ignore them or what they say about the enduring power of stigma.

On the very days of this meeting, in my home state, we are required to report on our application for a driver's license if we have ever been diagnosed with a "mental or emotional disorder" (Flynn, 1993). In 1994 a law came into effect requiring fingerprinting of all people identified as having a psychiatric diagnosis who come to any emergency treatment facility, emergency room, or are admitted to psychiatric units of general hospitals as well as all freestanding public and private psychiatric hospitals.

These manifestations of prejudice remain deeply disturbing to consumers and families alike. Nazi Germany may have passed into history half a century ago, but misinformation and discrimination are still alive and well (Beall, 1993a; Flynn, 1993).

We're haunted by the persistent, pernicious belief among too many treatment professionals that we're responsible for bringing these catastrophic disorders on ourselves, or on our children, by toxic parenting, moral dereliction, willful neglect, character weaknesses, or to use vernacular idiom, bad blood (Flynn, 1993).

We've rarely been viewed as capable of speaking for ourselves in any intelligent or intelligible way. To experience mental illness is to be incredibly devalued and dehumanized. In every sense possible, we have been, and too often still are, an abandoned, invisible, voiceless, powerless people (Beall, 1993a; Bevilacqua, 1992; Campbell & Frey, 1993; Peet, 1993).

As Laurie Flynn, director of the National Alliance for the Mentally Ill, said in her presentation, "With these disorders, with their history, with the second class status in medical care that many of our people are subject to and the fact that social control, limits on freedom, limits on responsibility have been such strong parts of the history for people with these disorders, there's a tremendous amount of suspicion about what it is you're really after when you talk about genetic counseling" (Flynn, 1993).

MY DOOR TO RECOVERY

Through all of the chaos and uncertainty some of us make it, more often by chance than by design. But we do recover. The unfortunate reality is that of the millions of people who experience major mental illness, only a tiny proportion of us have so far been able to access the kind and quality of care supportive of recovery (Beall, 1993b).

I'm going to tell you part of my story because of the critical role that my family history, and genetic information played in my understanding, and positive acceptance, of my psychiatric disabilities. How this happened opened the door to my active commitment to treatment and ultimately to recovery.

For the first time in my life, in these last years I've begun to trust there's life, real life, possible for me, despite major psychiatric disabilities. I can, for the first time, live with my mental illness not as a continuing cataclysm, but confident in the knowledge that I understand at least some of the factors that put me at risk for this particular disorder. I've seen PET scans of abnormal brain metabolism in others with my diagnosis. I know that effective treatment exists, good medications, behavioral and exposure therapies; I use them every day (Baxter, Schwartz, & Guze, 1991; Denkla, 1988; Zohar, Insel, & Rasmussen, 1991).

This knowledge and how it was offered to me made my recovery possible to the point where being a person with major mental illness is just another fact about me, like the color of my eyes, or my flair for graphic design.

There's a vast distinction between the acceptance we consumers experience when our mental disorders are presented to us by professionals as hideous life sentences from which there is no hope of reprieve, versus what is possible with informed acceptance and treatment partnerships for recovery. I've experienced both. One was immeasurably costly, one life restoring.

It seems almost diabolical that these illnesses strike in late adolescence and early adulthood right when other people are completing their training for chosen careers, marrying and founding families, while for people with major mental illness everything we hoped and dreamed and worked for is swept away.

There are no joyous school reunions for us. The smiles, the shared achievement, emphasize the unbearable gulf between our years of psychiatric hospitalizations, of hope, of promise never realized or realizable. It's been impossible to say to my peers that my advanced education equivalent is my psychiatric diagnosis and the crowning achievement of my life is that I'm still alive.

No one dreams of growing up to be mentally ill. It seems strange to talk of dreams, but the most exquisitely painful aspect of major mental illness was that it robbed me of all my dreams, of who I was, of who I might have been (Beall, 1993b).

Dreams seem so ephemeral, yet they lie at the heart of what it is to be human. Even more painfully, my illness stripped away the dreams of those I loved most, my family, my mother. To have no chance to achieve those dreams hurt worst of all.

The best metaphor for my illness is of being trapped inside a kaleidoscope. All of the familiar shapes and pieces of my life are in unexpected motion. I can at most times sense their familiarity but they're constantly shifting, sliding into new unknown configurations. My internal landscape is of change and unpredictability. Most of all I don't know how it will fall together ten minutes from now, no less a week from now. Or what terror I'll be gripped by, or who I'll be by then.

The very ground of my being was no longer secure.

Because we live in such internal uncertainty, walled about by such prejudice and misinformation, there is an intense hunger for concrete knowledge about our disorders among consumers. We yearn, we hunger for the truth, for information, for a humane, complete, and thorough education on every aspect of our illnesses. Not for another unproved theory of sociological or psychological etiology, we've been victimized by those too often, but an aching hunger for what can truly heal (Beall, 1993a).

We want to know everything, even if it is only fragmentary and at times uncertain or complex. We don't want truth to be packaged or sugarcoated. We want to be given both the certainty and the uncertainty (Beall, 1993a,b; Campbell & Schraiber, 1989).

Above all we need to know our disorders are real, that knowledge is out there, because we are desperate to find it and to draw on it. We know truth is the only substance from which we can reconstruct our lives. Truth, however hard, is the only path we know to recovery.

What's made these illnesses unspeakably grim is that we, who experience mental illness, like everyone else, have absorbed quite uncritically society's worst fears about crazies, wackos, insane ax murderers, and all the unreasoning prejudice and discrimination that surround the major mental illnesses.

How can I describe what we pass through when we begin to accept that we might be what society thinks we are, with all of the frightful myths, the bizarre assumptions, as we finally give up and feel out that horrifying shape in its multiple dimensions.

Many years ago I'd no choice but to accept how little of my behavior was under my control. Accept that I no longer knew from day to day, or hour to hour, who I was, or what I might be driven to do.

There is nothing that can prepare one for the reality of major mental illness. We have no positive models of how to do it with grace, or style. No one takes on major mental illness to get attention or to rebel. There are many, far more effective and interesting ways to do that, starting, as the old song goes, with "sex and drugs and rock and roll."

My earliest memory as a tiny child is of being driven to pick up sharp objects, pieces of metal, shards of glass. I believed that if I didn't, someone would be hurt, cut, or killed because I didn't get rid of all the possibly hurtful things. That I, through my negligence, would be responsible for catastrophic harm coming to people I didn't even know.

Gradually I became convinced I was responsible for all of the harm that came to anyone, anywhere—a large burden for so small a child.

To distance myself from any power to hurt or harm, I spoke for years only in the third person.

Even after I realized I was different from everyone else in frightening ways, I still believed that as I grew into the authority and power of adulthood I'd finally be able to be like everyone else. But as I grew, the disorder grew, both in complexity and in power.

I collected all the sharp things I could find, on the ground, in the road, in vacant lots, and stashed them in the back of my clothes closet. My mother, who lived in terror of contamination and contagion, who washed her hands until they were like cracked bleeding sandpaper, eradicated the evidence of my safety campaign each morning the instant I was safely ensconced on the school bus headed down the mountain toward Athens.

I was gripped by counting and touching rituals. To go through a door I had to tap my feet a certain way, or touch and tap the walls. My sister could only eat food in a certain order and only if nothing on her plate touched anything else.

My mother quite literally followed me around the apartment with a cloth in her hand, cleaning everything I touched. Not just any cleaning rag, but a cloth she made of double-sided flannel, which she hemmed by hand in a very special way, with a specific stitch, done perfectly. We lived in rural Greece at the end of a civil war and two-sided flannel wasn't easy to come by.

If I couldn't complete my rituals I was consumed by terror. If I couldn't do a specific warding motion, or series of calculations, or mental gymnastics, my feelings of impeding catastrophe became so overwhelming, I could hardly keep in touch with what was happening around me.

As I grew older I learned to use the bathroom, or a refuge on the mountainside where I'd be alone to do the rituals I couldn't disguise as something socially acceptable. I very quickly learned to be the complete loner.

School became my personal horror show. In the end, even though I've some gift of intelligence, the pure intellectual obsessions held knowledge hostage. And so I lost learning, which I love as much as life itself.

I spent my adult life searching for effective treatment. For years I tried talking therapies and medications with no appreciable positive result. I continued to experience the same severe symptoms I always had, but in addition I suffered terrible and humiliating side effects from the medications. I lost control of my bladder, I could not see, my heart did not work right, and my original symptoms continued unabated.

I believe the professionals who were trying to help me genuinely liked me. It was as hard on them as it was on me that nothing anyone tried worked. Little by little they began to ask if my symptoms couldn't possibly be my way of capturing and holding their attention.

I felt sick and truly afraid. The very people to whom I'd entrusted the most intimate secrets from the depths of my soul felt I wasn't trying to get well. The people who I thought were the experts believed I didn't want to get well, that I chose to be sick, and that's why I didn't get better. I was gripped by despair.

I didn't know how to try harder, so I gave up. I lost all hope for myself. I tried living with my disorder without all the side effects. I quit medication. I quit talking. I withdrew from all social contact except that absolutely necessary for survival.

I lived with the terror, the rituals, with constant "static" of rhymes and music running in endless circles in my brain. I isolated myself and saw others only when I was able to "pass."

In the consumer community those of us who are middle-aged or older are the survivors of what I've come to call the Etiology Wars. Please understand, as I tell you my story, that my goal is *not* to criticize the many professionals who gave their working lives to helping people like me. My purpose is rather to examine how we, patients and professionals alike, coped with the age-old mystery of mental illness in the absence of hard knowledge, with only well-meaning theories to guide us.

Good people searched with pathetically inadequate tools for any clue, any understanding, any possible answer. As they tried out theory after theory, people like me were those on whom all the unsuccessful theories were tried, one after the other.

There were so many competing theories, uncertainty in diagnoses, such varying schools of thought. As a consumer in the middle of it all I was swamped. Each school of thought had its own arcane explanation for mental illness, its own ideology of cure. Professionals and academics squabbled with each other over details of etiology in ways that sounded uncomfortably like obscure doctrinal feuds among medieval monks. All I know is, I tried them all, and all of them failed.

To allow myself to hope again became impossible in the face of so much unrelieved failure. It just hurt too much, I gave up on treatment of any kind. I chose to live with the continuous unrelievable pressure of impending, unimaginable catastrophe, the terror, the rituals, the nonsense sounds and music running endlessly in my brain even when I slept. I hunkered down and settled for bare survival.

My husband has major depression. We met in high school and both of us went away to college only to find ourselves disintegrating. We married in our first year of college and provided for each other a lifeline, a haven we could never have survived without. The blessing of our marriage is that we were never profoundly ill at the same time. To be mentally ill, and to survive, one needs a champion on the outside who will fight ceaselessly for your life.

Ray's experience with treatment was different from mine. He'd had a devastating bout of depression early in his freshman year which he survived without major interventions. The next year after we were married it returned. He sat day after day in the living room facing a corner, hunched over, tears running silently on his face.

I got him to a student health service psychologist who urged him to withdraw from school, but strongly advised me to try to wait out the depression without turning Ray over to a public mental health hospital, because he might well be hospitalized indefinitely. That was how it was done then, in rural Ohio.

I froze in place, gripped by certain terror I was responsible for what was happening to Ray. Somehow through multiple bouts of paralyzing depression he made it through college. We learned to suffer and to stubbornly endure.

After Ray graduated he put himself in the care of the director of a famous analytic institute. The most I can say for those grim years was Ray managed to emerge from them alive. For a young struggling family the cost of analysis meant used clothes for our children, a single pair of shoes at a time, and the end of any hope I had of advanced education.

Finally the analyst died. Ray turned to our internist for advice and was referred to a very competent psychopharmacologist who put him on the oldest of the MAOIs, an antidepressant available, if only he had known it, for over 35 years.

In 2 weeks he was the man I had met and fallen in love with a quarter of a century before. He was, however, in the iron grip of grief and rage.

He felt he'd been imprisoned needlessly in the depths of depression by a bad treatment decision to which he was never privy. He'd been condemned to struggle hopelessly for years believing he was at fault, missing his children's growing years, the possibility of fully developing the promise of his talents and frozen developmentally in his teens, the age when the depression became intractable. As he says with a sweet bitter smile, "I'm 50 going on 17." Worst of all he came to learn that analysis could never have worked alone to lift depression of the severity he experienced.

In all those years of talking and suffering, he'd never been offered the knowledge by the professionals treating him that there were any other choices for treatment.

I was full of joy and relief for him, but jealous, too. I was possessed by the notion that he had recovered because he had tried harder and somehow was a better person, more worthy than I. I feared and loathed myself for the moral weakness at the core of my being I'd come to accept as the cause of my mental illness.

Right there is the seductive core of psychotherapy. Being dependent on a prescription for one's sanity has been made to seem the depths of moral dereliction to our addiction-phobic society, the ultimate lack of spine and character.

The notion that if one digs deep enough in the back closets of the soul, you can cure yourself by solving an intricate internal puzzle of symbol and shadow, to emerge stronger and better is powerfully seductive. So too is a promise of cure not dependent on drugs or the humiliation of a body racked by medication side effects. Don't we all wish it were that easy.

But it isn't. Talking can't cure severe psychiatric disabilities, not schizophrenia, or manic-depression, or severe anxiety, or obsessive-compulsive disorder, or panic, or the other major mental illnesses. But, oh my, how much suffering and damage analysts and other true believers have inflicted on people like us!

My daughter, Edith, and my husband, Ray, never gave up on me. They kept faith with the woman they loved, and in whose existence I no longer believed.

My daughter has a refractory form of epilepsy, and some years ago, long after I'd given up in despair, her neurologist announced that I'd been misdiagnosed. I didn't just have major depression, but also a severe anxiety disorder and OCD.

I wasn't convinced. I'd closed the door on treatment.

For 9 months Ray and Edith pressed me on a daily basis until I finally gave in and made an appointment to see the doctor the neurologist recommended. I went on the condition that if I saw this doctor once they would get out of my face and never bring the subject up again.

I stalked into his office and snarled that I was coerced into seeing him, that my family would not get off my case until I saw him once, but that I didn't believe in treatment.

He replied that if he couldn't help me, he was indeed the wrong person and I shouldn't come back. I was stunned. He listened to me, and spoke to me as an equal. He explained he had experience in treating hundreds of people like me, but I was the sole expert on my disorder and my symptoms.

He explained in detail what obsessive-compulsive disorder was. He showed me pictures of brain scans of people with OCD. He went over all its symptoms and all the different ways it manifests itself. He explained what was known about its genetics.

He drew a chart of my family and did a careful analysis of my extended family and his understanding of genetics and its complexities. As I sat there

I remembered my mother speaking of her aunt and how Nannie committed suicide the week I was born. So many facts clicked together in my brain. It finally all made sense.

I almost couldn't take it in. What had the power to reach me as nothing else, was the stunning realization that my own mother, reclusive, terrified of germs and contamination of any kind, suffered the same disorder I did. It manifested itself in a different symptom set. The doctor wrote a prescription and asked me to return for at least three more visits.

He gave me articles and a bibliography (Andreasen, 1984; Baxter *et al.,* 1991; Denkla, 1988; Jenike, Baer, & Minicheillo, 1986; Rapoport, 1989; Zohar *et al.,* 1991).

I stumbled out of my chair. He made me sit back down. He didn't want me to leave his office confused or overwhelmed.

I went home and cried for days. I had to wash all that hideous useless treatment history away before I could go forward.

What made the difference? Certainly information about my family history was critically important, but also his absolute honesty about what was *not* known, and its uncertainties. It was as much what he knew as how he interacted with me, his personal commitment to treating me as a full human being, and working with me as an equal partner.

My recovery began then, at that moment (Spaniol & Kechler, 1994).

He taught me what he'd learned from his other patients about how I might be able to control my mental illness. He gave me the opportunity to try out a variety of strategies to control my symptoms. This way I learned what works and what doesn't for me. He gave control of my life, and my mental illness, back to me.

In a matter of weeks my most troubling symptoms were responding to treatment. After a lifetime of terrible struggle, suffering, and hiding, for the first time in my life I could be normal. I could begin again, leave all the suffering behind me.

A CLOSING NOTE

In the end I came to understand that the very fabric of who I am was forged in the crucible of mental illness. I can't walk away. Not from myself. Not from other consumers who I've come to love and respect. I can't walk away from those still trapped in the grips of their disorders. People needing more courage than most of us can imagine, just to pick up and keep trying again and again each and every day. There's no way I'd leave them behind. I want them to have the same chance to recover I've had. Even if that means reconfiguring and retooling the public treatment system so it can deliver quality care, and positive measurable outcomes.

Consumers and families can't do this enormous job alone. Only when research professionals and treatment professionals unite with us will we be able to push this cruelly dysfunctional treatment system into change. It will take all of us working together.

How geneticists and other research scientists frame new information will be decisive in how it's used, and if it will be used in humane ways to do humane things. In this technologically oriented society they have the gift of unusual power to get and hold attention, the authority to command respect (Beall, 1993b; Flynn, 1993).

Real systems change will take place when our combined voices tell the truth, even if we must say the current public system doesn't work, that the emperor has no clothes. To build anew we must name what doesn't work and can never work (Bevilacqua, 1992; Blanch, 1992; Campbell & Frey, 1993; Penny, 1993; Shamoo & Irving, 1993).

Paul, before he died, made me promise to write my story and place it where it could be read and understood by researchers and professionals. My most powerful obsession, with which I've wrestled every day of my life, made it impossible for me to put pencil to paper, and write about or share my internal world shaped by mental illnesses. The hardest thing we ever did was the work we began together, to overcome it.

His brilliant grasp of the genetic and neurobiological factors in mental illness convinced me to trust him enough to take up the fight for my life once again, in the midst of despair and what felt like coercion.

More than a doctor, he was a gifted healer who fought suffering at every turn, a patient teacher who taught me how to recover hope, dignity, and life itself. Most of all he encouraged me. Celebrated my victories. He modeled respect, the moral use of power, the very best of what it is to be human. Because I could trust him, I learned again how to trust myself.

With loving respect, I dedicate this chapter to the memory of Dr. Lon Paul Travis, M.D. I was never able to thank him for what he did, for who he was. My most profound prayer is that there are others of his kind in the world for people like me to find.

REFERENCES

Andreasen, N. (1984). *The broken brain.* New York: Harper & Row.
Baxter, L. R., Schwartz, J. M., & Guze, B. H. (1991). Brain imaging: Toward a neuroanatomy of obsessive-compulsive disorder. In J. Zohar, T. Insel, & S. Rasmussen (Eds.), *The psychobiology of obsessive-compulsive disorder.* Berlin: Springer.
Beall, M. A. (1993a). *Virginia Mental Health Consumers Association Commissioners Guidance Questionnaire: Survey Results November 1992.* Richmond: Virginia Mental Health Consumers Association.
Beall, M. A. (1993b). President, Virginia Mental Health Consumers Association, Member of

the Board of Directors NAMI, remarks at "Understanding the Role of Genetic Factors in Mental Illness: Bridging the Gap Between Research and Society," a workshop sponsored by the Office of Technology Assessment and the National Institute of Mental Health, January 21–23, 1993.

Bevilacqua, J. J. (1992). South Carolina Commissioner of Mental Health, Columbia, SC. "Consummerism and the Mental Health System: An Elusive Relationship." Keynote address. Annual Southern Regional Conference on Mental Health Statistics, New Orleans, September 28, 1992.

Biesecker, B. B. (1993). National Center for Human Genome Research, National Institutes of Health, Bethesda, MD, remarks at "Understanding the Role of Genetic Factors in Mental Illness: Bridging the Gap Between Research and Society," a workshop sponsored by the Office of Technology Assessment and the National Institute of Mental Health, January 21–23, 1993.

Blanch, A. (1992). *Proceedings of Roundtable Discussion on the Use of Involuntary Interventions: Multiple Perspectives.* Rockville, MD: Community Support Program Center for Mental Health Services.

Campbell, J., & Frey, E. D. (1993). *Humanizing decision support systems.* Rockville, MD: Mental Health Statistical Improvement Program, Center for Mental Health Services.

Campbell, J., Ralph, R., & Glover, R. (1994). *From lab rat to researcher: Policy implications of consumer/survivor involvement in research.* Alexandria, VA: National Association of State Mental Health Program Directors Research Institute.

Campbell, J., & Schraiber, R. (1989). *The Well-Being Project: Mental health clients speak for themselves* (Vol. 6). Sacramento: California Department of Mental Health.

Clements, M. (1993, October 31). What we say about mental illness. *Parade Magazine,* pp. 4–6.

Cook-Deegan, R. M. (1993). Remarks at "Understanding the Role of Genetic Factors in Mental Illness: Bridging the Gap Between Research and Society," a workshop sponsored by the Office of Technology Assessment and the National Institute of Mental Health, January 21–23, 1993.

Coursey, R. D., Farrell, D. W., & Zahniser, J. H. (1991). Consumer attitudes towards psychotherapy, hospitalization and aftercare. *Health and Social Work, 16,* 155–161.

Denkla, M. B. (1988). Neurological examination. In J. L. Rapoport (Ed.), *Obsessive-compulsive disorder in children and adolescents.* Washington, DC: American Psychiatric Press.

Diamond, R. J., & Factor, R. M. (1994, March). Taking issue. *Hospital and Community Psychiatry, 45,* No. 3.

Flynn, L. (1993). Executive Director, National Alliance for the Mentally Ill, Arlington, VA, remarks at "Understanding the Role of Genetic Factors in Mental Illness: Bridging the Gap Between Research and Society," a workshop sponsored by the Office of Technology Assessment and the National Institute of Mental Health, January 21–23, 1993.

Folstein, S. (1993). Johns Hopkins, Baltimore, MD, remarks at "Understanding the Role of Genetic Factors in Mental Illness: Bridging the Gap Between Research and Society," a workshop sponsored by the Office of Technology Assessment and the National Institute of Mental Health, January 21–23, 1993.

Gershon, E. (1993). Chief of Clinical Neurogenetics, National Institute of Mental Health, Bethesda, MD, remarks at "Understanding the Role of Genetic Factors in Mental Illness: Bridging the Gap Between Research and Society," a workshop sponsored by the Office of Technology Assessment and the National Institute of Mental Health, January 21–23, 1993.

Gottesman, I. I. (1991). *Schizophrenia genesis: The origins of madness.* San Francisco: Freeman.

Green, C. (1994, September 11). I know there is help. *Parade Magazine,* pp. 4–8.

Jenike, M. A., Baer, L., & Minicheillo, W. E. (Eds.). (1986). *Obsessive-compulsive disorders: Theory and management.* Littleton, MA: PSG Publishing.

Marsh, D. T. (Ed.). (1994). *New directions in the psychological treatment of serious mental illness.* Westport, CT: Praeger.

Pardes, H. (1993). Workshop Chair, College of Physicians and Surgeons, Columbia University, New York, remarks at "Understanding the Role of Genetic Factors in Mental Illness: Bridging the Gap Between Research and Society," a workshop sponsored by the Office of Technology Assessment and the National Institute of Mental Health, January 21–23, 1993.

Peavey, D. L. (1994). *Ethical dilemmas of the consumer/professional.* Anchorage, AK: 101 East Ninth Ave. #3A.

Peet, M. J. (1993). Deputy Commissioner of Mental Health, Connecticut Department of Mental Health. "Oppression Holds Back Everyone." Keynote address. Conference on Consumers as Mental Health Staff, New Haven, CT, November 3, 1993.

Penny, D. (Ed.). (1993). *Preliminary thoughts on best practices for establishing state offices of consumer/ex-patient affairs.* Holyoke, MA: Human Resource Association.

Rapoport, J. L. (1989). *The boy who couldn't stop washing.* New York: Dutton.

Rodgers, W. H., Wells, K., Merideth, L., & Sturm, R. (1993). Outcomes for adults with depression under pre paid or fee for service financing. *Archives of General Psychiatry, 50,* 517–525.

Sapers, B. (1994). Harvard Medical School Student, remarks at Research Plenary, Carol Reese, "The good news: Research, funds, technology for neuroscientists." *NAMI Advocate,* Vol. 16, No. 1.

Shamoo, A. E., & Irving, D. N. (1993). Accountability in research using persons with mental illness. *Accountability in Research, 3,* 1–17.

Spaniol, L., & Kechler, M. (Eds.). (1994). *The experience of recovery.* Boston: Center for Pscyhiatric Rehabilitation.

Tanzman, B. H. (1990). *Researching the preference of people with psychiatric disabilities for housing and supports: A practical guide.* Burlington, VT: Center for Community Change Through Housing and Supports.

Trochim, W., Dumont, J., & Campbell, J. (1993). *Mapping mental health outcomes from the perspective of consumer/survivors.* Alexandria, VA: National Association of State Mental Health Program Directors Research Institute, Inc.

Tsuang, M. T. (1993). Harvard School of Medicine, Cambridge, MA, remarks at "Understanding the Role of Genetic Factors in Mental Illness: Bridging the Gap Between Research and Society," a workshop sponsored by the Office of Technology Assessment and the National Institute of Mental Health, January 21–23, 1993.

Weiden, P. (1994). St. Lukes–Roosevelt Hospital Center, New York. "Medication Noncompliance in Schizophrenia: A Public Health Problem." Delivered at the Convention of the National Alliance for the Mentally Ill, San Antonio, TX, July 1994.

Zohar, J., Insel, T. R., & Rasmussen, S. (Eds.). (1991). *The psychobiology of obsessive-compulsive disorder.* Berlin: Springer.

CHAPTER 8

The Human Implications of Psychiatric Genetics

LAURA LEE HALL

Research involves people. People participate in research. People may bene-fit from research-driven improvements in clinical practice. And people face social perceptions and policies that stem from research.

Study of the genetic factors involved in mental disorders is no different. However, the polemics and controversy surrounding the genetics of mental disorders forestall reasoned discussion of what this research means to peo-ple with mental disorders and their families. The complexity of this research further compounds consideration of its clinical and social implications. And the uncertainty of the genetic mechanisms involved in mental disorders deters many from spending time (or money) on this topic.

It may be unwise to devote a great deal of time and resources to the consideration of specific policies and implications of the genetics of mental disorders, given the early stage of research findings. But no discussion also seems an unwise choice. Clinicians, policymakers, people with mental disorders and their family members are left to decipher the complicated, confusing, and unevenly reported research results. No discussion also means that little opportunity for interdisciplinary dialogue exists among geneticists, mental health professionals, genetic counselors, ethicists, social analysts,

This chapter is adapted from Hall, L. L. (1994). Implications for society. In *Mental Disorders and Genetics: Bridging the Gap between Research and Society.* U.S. Congress, Office of Technol-ogy Assessment, OTA-BP-H-133. Washington, DC: Government Printing Office.

LAURA LEE HALL • National Alliance for the Mentally Ill, Arlington, Virginia 22203.
Genetics and Mental Illness: Evolving Issues for Research and Society, edited by Laura Lee Hall. Plenum Press, New York, 1996.

people with mental disorders and their family members and friends. People have no formal venue for voicing their concerns; experts outside of the mental health field have no official forum in which to share their experiences and knowledge.

A workshop hosted by the Office of Technology Assessment (OTA), an analytical support agency for the U.S. Congress, and the National Institute of Mental Health (NIMH) in January of 1993 provided one of the first opportunities for comprehensive discourse of the issues raised specifically by genetic studies of mental disorders. Experts within and outside of the mental health field, as well as consumer representatives, discussed ethical issues that emerge during this research, the clinical implications of what we know about the genetics of mental disorders, and how society views these topics. The panel's deliberations evinced the concerns many have about the genetics of mental disorders and characterized issues that have already emerged. This chapter documents the workshop discussion under three headings:

- Ethics and research
- Genetic counseling
- Public perceptions and social implications

ETHICS AND RESEARCH

Diagnostic and treatment advances result from research, including studies involving human subjects. While few question the value of biomedical research in general, publicized abuses over the course of the 20th century highlight the need to safeguard the rights and well-being of research participants. Research of the genetic factors involved in mental disorders is no different; protection of research participants is a preeminent concern. However, the necessary involvement of whole families, the stigma and discrimination attached to genetic and mental disorders, and the potential impact of mental disorders on reasoning and judgment compound and complicate ethical concerns. Workshop participants elaborated some of the difficult ethical issues that emerge from this research. In addition, several participants signaled the need for guidance on how to better deal with these situations.

The ethical conduct of research involving human subjects rests on a bedrock of three values, first enumerated by the National Commission for the Protection of Human Subjects of Biomedical and Behavioral Research (National Commission): respect for persons, beneficence, and justice (Murray, 1993; U.S. Congress, 1993; U.S. Department of Health, Education and Welfare 1978). Respect allows people to make and pursue their own decisions in an informed and voluntary manner. Beneficence seeks both to protect individuals from harm and to ensure benefits from research involving human subjects. Justice refers to the fair and uncoerced selection of human subjects for research, especially among vulnerable populations.

The regulatory translation of these ethical principles guides nearly all research with human subjects today. Specifically, federal regulations demand that all federally funded human research projects must be reviewed and approved by an Institutional Review Board or IRB ([45 CFR 46.103(b)]. This multidisciplinary panel considers risks, benefits, subject selection, and other issues for proposed studies involving human subjects. Federal regulations further require that informed consent be obtained from each subject, although this can be waived in certain circumstances. In order to provide informed consent, the anticipated benefits and potential risks associated with an experimental procedure must be explained to the individual; he or she must understand these factors, rationally weigh them, and then make a voluntary decision as to whether or not to participate.

Informed consent, while straightforward in principle, can be challenging to obtain, especially in complicated research designs. Packed with technical information, lengthy, or even incomplete, consent forms may baffle all but those with specialized expertise. One workshop panelist described this concern and the need for one-on-one, ongoing discussion to achieve informed consent (Biesecker, 1993):

> We now have a pretty impressive informed consent form for breast cancer genetic research after a lot of work ... on two single spaced typed pages. Academically, we may have finally thought through many issues and anticipated some of them. But how do potential participants process all this and make a decision for themselves that they want to or do not want to participate in this research? ... Our most successful endeavors have been engaging individuals in one-one-one conversations. ... True informed consent is a discussion and a long, ongoing process.

Although never translated into regulation, the National Commission acknowledged that mental disorders, which impact on cognitive processes, emotions, and behavior, may sometimes impair the ability to provide informed consent (U.S. Congress, 1993). The limited research data that exist fortify this observation. Severe symptoms of schizophrenia, including psychosis, paranoia, or delusions, can compromise an individual's competence to provide informed consent (Grisso & Appelbaum, 1991; P. A. Appelbaum, personal communication, July 11, 1994).

Of course, if a person is found incompetent to provide informed consent, proxy consent, given by a legally authorized representative, may be required and under certain circumstances requirements for informed consent may be waived (Shore et al., 1993). However, these approaches to consent are unlikely to be used commonly. For one, even hospitalized individuals with schizophrenia exhibit a considerable range of capacities to provide informed consent (Grisso & Appelbaum, 1991). And as one panelist noted, IRBs around the country may not be informed on this subject (Shore, 1993):

> A meeting held recently, jointly sponsored by the Office for Protection from Research Risks, the National Center for Human Genome Research, and NIMH, . . . found that institutionwide IRBs know relatively little about mental disorders and they may need to be better informed about consent issues, substituted judgment issues and the like.

Perhaps most importantly, people with mental disorders and their families urge greater participation in research (Flynn, 1993):

> I'm not at all certain that we have done all that we can or the best job we could in terms of really thinking appropriately about informed consent. I appreciate the difficulties and understand the concerns that people have about the impact on the research enterprise, but I also think that we have to respect what others are telling us about the increasing role that consumers are playing in their own lives and in shaping their own lives. My own information that we gather from talking to people in our office is that the work that's done is focused on getting a signature. Get the signature, get the paper signed. Sometimes there's a good description and discussion of what's going on and what may occur and what the research is pointing towards and sometimes it's not so good and not so thorough.
>
> In almost all cases it occurs once. I think we need to realize particularly in research of this type that we may want to see it as less an event and more a process. We may want to be sure as the research unfolds that those people most directly involved and affected continue to be updated and advised and understand what, in fact, is going on.
>
> So I think we need to think more comprehensively about a partnership with the people who are involved as research subjects and recognize there's a lot more to consent than getting someone who is now not under the protection of some of the rest of the field because they are specifically excluded. . . . There is some unfinished business in that regard. I think we need to be particularly sensitive to respecting our duty to inform and perhaps inform more than one way more than one time so that people can be full participants and partners in the research.

The conclusions of the workshop discussants—that informed consent requires more than a one-time paper signing event, that the issue of mental disorders and informed consent must be taken seriously, and that IRBs require support and education—echo the findings of a recent report from the Office for the Protection from Research Risks (OPRR)[1] (Frankel & Teich, 1993; U.S. Department of Health and Human Services, 1993). Panel-

---

[1]The office is located in the National Institute of Health, U.S. Department of Health and Human Services.

ists also urged greater sensitivity to the families of participants in research (Honberg, 1993):

> In mental illness the research subjects may be fairly young ... between the ages of 18 and 21 ... with serious mental illness, and the families may be very involved in the individual's life.... I would maintain in that type of situation ... that the ... ethical obligation (for informed consent and ongoing communication) extends to the family as well.
>
> Let me give you an example. Say a family has identified a particular research protocol at a particular university and has informed the individual who has the mental illness of that program and they've made a collective decision that that program is an appropriate one and the individual goes to the program and at some point sits down and is informed about the research protocol and the risks of the research and the potential benefits of the research, et cetera.
>
> In that type of situation where there is no apparent disagreement between the individual and his or her family, it would be my contention and I believe it's NAMI's (National Alliance for the Mentally Ill) contention that the obligation on the part of the researchers to inform would extend to the family. In other words, they would have an obligation to sit down with the family as well as that individual.
>
> I realize that I just introduced a new subject, but that's something that we hear about a great deal, that families initiate a referral and then they're completely written out of the process.

Several panelists expressed the opinion that family members should be more involved in research, participating in the consent process, in ongoing contact with researchers, and as members of IRBs (Beall, 1993; Cox, 1993). In pedigree studies, families are necessary participants, which challenges the traditional vantage point of bioethics. Concern for the individual subjects has directed the evolution of bioethical concepts of informed consent, confidentiality, and voluntary participation. Researchers and ethicists on our panel noted the difficulties of adapting these ethical principles to studies involving whole families. One such issue raised by genetic research and discussed at the workshop is disputed paternity (Conneally, 1993):

> I feel privacy must be breached ... in situations involving disputed paternity. I've had two cases where two daughters of two different individuals thought they were at risk for Huntington's when in fact they were not. That brings up two points. Obviously, they were told, in fact, in one case I had to tell the individual because the mother would not. In the other, the mother did eventually, after a lot of arm twisting, tell the daughter that, in fact she was not at risk. In both cases, these two young women were pregnant. Now, that creates another issue and you might argue that the mother' privacy shouldn't be breached, but I feel that there's a right—that the daughter has a right to know something that impacts on the rest of her life, just as well as her mother has a right not to have anyone know what she did some 20 years earlier.

As the above example illustrates, pedigree research can reveal previously unshared information about biological relationships among family
members. Such information pits the rights of some family members to their
privacy against the rights of others to know if they or their children are at
increased risk for a condition. Although researchers worry about discom-
forting and discouraging would-be research participants, several panelists
gave voice to the opinion that pedigree research's ability to expose disputed
paternity is required for true informed consent (Cox, 1993; Murray, 1993):

> In discussing the business about informed consent, it's clear that unless that
> potential is brought out, one could be accused of violating the ethical principle
> of informed consent. In other words, if that's a possibility—even a relatively
> low risk—it must be revealed. And it's not relatively low, it's relatively high.
> In some communities that I deal with, it's not five percent, it's more like 15 or
> 20 percent. . . . There are two ways of dealing with it. One is to have this in the
> informed consent form, and the other is to take the pedigree by asking, "Is this
> man the father of all your children?" [Murray, 1993].

Disputed paternity is not the only aspect of pedigree research that
may incur conflict among family members. The very issue of informed
consent becomes more complex, as described by one workshop participant
(Cook-Deegan, 1993):

> One of the things that is unique about pedigree studies is the fact that it's no
> longer a dyadic relationship between a patient and a person involved in a clinical
> trial or other research. There are other people involved in the family. Does
> every person on that pedigree have to have an informed consent statement
> before you publish it? Do you publish it? How much clinical information do
> you include? Should you alter the pedigree to prevent identification? All these
> questions about how to handle the information in pedigree research are being
> raised without much inspection except by the ethical norms of the people doing it.

Not only does a single individual consent to participate in a pedigree
study, but the participant must be informed that relatives will be asked to
participate (Shore *et al.,* 1993; U.S. Department of Health and Human
Services, 1993). Family members participating in the study must be given
the option to consent as well. Researchers must decide and inform participants of which information will be shared with family participants. A medical geneticist and ethicist on the workshop panel noted (Murray, 1993):

> Most IRBs I am familiar with . . . treat the pedigree as part of the patient record
> and therefore all the information related to that patient is considered confidential
> in the same way that clinical records are considered confidential. They don't
> approach any other members of the family for testing unless they get the permis-
> sion from the proband or consultant in the pedigree.

Of course, problems can emerge if family members disagree about participation in a research project. An example from research in Huntington's disease is illustrative (Conneally, 1993):

> A young woman completed a Family History Questionnaire and signed an informed consent form placing her family on the Roster. When asked to identify family members who would be best suited to complete an affected questionnaire, she identified her brother. A packet of information concerning Huntington's disease and explaining the purpose of the Affected Questionnaire was sent to the brother. Several days after the questionnaire was mailed, a certified letter from the brother's attorney was received stating that he wanted "his family" removed from the Roster.

Family members may have different feelings about a disease or about participating in research. Individuals may want to ignore the presence of a disease within their family, deny its existence, or may guard such information as a secret, even from other family members. Stigmatized genetic conditions and mental disorders are certainly sensitive issues for many families. These concerns highlight the unique kinds of risks that pedigree studies pose to individuals and families. While physical risks, such as possible side effects of a new medication, may be minimal or nonexistent in pedigree research, information about genetic status or mental disorder pose what a recent OPRR report calls *psychosocial risks.* "Information can provoke anxiety and confusion, damage familial relationships, and compromise a subject's insurability and employment opportunities" (U.S. Department of Health and Human Services, 1993). IRBs may not appreciate the nature of these risks and thus may dismiss them as insignificant, a neglect that OPRR cautions against.

Because of the psychosocial risks presented by genetic research, confidentiality of information becomes paramount. Experts advise that as much information as possible be kept private from other family members participating in genetic studies. Information that must be revealed should be disclosed only with the full knowledge and agreement of each participant. But privacy or confidentiality concerns extend beyond family members. Family and genetic studies of mental disorders can unearth a host of sensitive information, such as the presence of a mental disorder, increased family risk for a condition, other behavioral problems, substance abuse, and criminal history. This type of information in the hands of private insurers, employers, or others could pose grave risks to an individual participating in research. To address this concern, NIMH encourages the use of certificates of confidentiality to prevent access to individually identifiable research data by insurance companies, government authorities, or other third parties. Evolved in the context of substance abuse research, this

certificate protects investigators from the compulsory revelation of potentially harmful research data (42 CFR Part 2a, 1991). Indeed, an NIMH
scientist indicated that the mental health research community increasingly
uses certificates of confidentiality (Shore, 1993).

The certificate of confidentiality does not preclude reporting cases of
child abuse or imminent suicidal or homicidal behavior. Neither does the
certificate of confidentiality inoculate against the inadvertent revelation of
information by the research subject, as noted at the meeting (Shore, 1993):

> Let me warn you that there's a potential leak in the system. Not so much in
> the system, but in the way in which it's used practically. Individuals who go for
> testing before they enter a research protocol may be told, "Well, we'll be happy
> to enter you in our protocol, but we need to be sure about the diagnosis. We
> need to have certain blood tests," and the person goes in to their private physician
> and says, "I want to get a blood test to check out X, Y, and Z, and the reason
> is that I'm about to participate in a research study on the genetics of Alzheimer's
> disease." So, the physician writes down, "To participate in research study on
> Alzheimer's disease, ordering the following tests," and files for insurance reim-
> bursement. The person himself has already let out of the bag information which
> can and will go to the insurance company.

Apprising research participants about this potential problem is yet
another important component of informed consent. Finally, F. D. Burgmann (personal communication, July 30, 1994), a representative from The
National Depressive and Manic-Depressive Association notes that:

> [a] Confidentiality Statement serves no purpose if the storage of research data
> is accessible. Any data storage device that has telecommunication ability, or
> that is networked to such a main server is vulnerable. ALL RESEARCH DATA
> WITH ANY FORM OF PATIENT IDENTIFIER, INCLUDING "INTER-
> NAL CODE," MUST BE ISOLATED DURING WORK AND KEPT IN
> A STAND-ALONE DATA BASE WITH NO TELECOMMUNICATION
> INTERFACE AT ALL [capitalization in original letter]. We feel this is abso-
> lutely necessary, absolutely imperative to protect information from incursion
> by 1) government at any level, 2) insurance companies, 3) current or prospective
> employers, 4) media snoops, 5) current or prospective family members, and 6)
> hackers. Should the research data for any particular individual be requested
> that patient should be asked to execute a specific Release of Information.

While not discussed in great detail, workshop participants also raised
concerns about how to handle data and biological materials after a research
subject withdraws from a study or in future studies, for which informed
consent was not specifically garnered. Federal regulations clearly require
that subjects be free to withdraw from a research project without penalty
or loss of benefits to which they are otherwise entitled. Regulations do not
address the use of data or tissue samples should a participant decline further
study participation. A panelist noted that the ruling in a 1990 California

Supreme Court case—*John Moore v. The Regents of the University of California*—provides guidance (Shore, 1993). In that case, the court held that cell lines transformed from a donated blood sample are not the property of the person who donated the sample. In line with this ruling, workshop participants speculated that people who withdraw from a genetic research project might not necessarily be able to require destruction of all of the information and biological materials previously provided. There are questions about this case's applicability, however. For example, could a withdrawing research subject request that all identifiers linking the data or samples to him or her be purged? Also, *Moore* constitutes binding legal authority only in California. As of this writing, it has not been adopted in other jurisdictions.

Having invested considerable time and resources into the collection of data and biological materials from extended families, researchers may desire to test new genetic markers or hypotheses as they arise. Must researchers seek renewed informed consent? Most experts do not advise the destruction of valuable and perhaps irreplaceable resources. On the other hand, relevant ethical concerns raised by a new study may make renewed informed consent indispensable. A Huntington's disease researcher described his approach to this problem (Conneally, 1993):

> I would be concerned if I collected DNA on people and then simply discarded it when it might be very useful to them. So I would suggest that you have an informed consent saying that we're going to keep this DNA and it will only be used with your written consent, like we do in our Huntington's disease DNA bank.

OPRR offers similar guidance (U.S. Department of Health an Human Services, 1993):

> Where a new study proposes to use samples collected for a previously conducted study, IRBs should consider whether the consent given for the earlier study also applies to the new study. Where the purposes of the new study diverge significantly from the purposes of the original protocol, and where the new study depends on the familial identifiability of the samples, new consent should be obtained.

What if research results become clinically relevant? Should someone be informed if it becomes clear that he or she has a 90% risk of developing a serious medical disorder, for which preventive interventions or effective therapies exist? Several obstacles preclude a simple yes in response to this question. An individual who participates in research may not want to know such information. A researcher in a laboratory, who has had no contact with the subject, may make the health risk discovery. In this situation, who contacts the research subject? Researchers assert that the question should be put to subjects directly: if we discover that you are at risk for a severe disease which is preventable, do you want us to inform you? NIMH's approach to this topic offers one example. It advises its grantees that consent documents clearly indicate whether subjects will be given the results of genetic tests used in research (Shore *et al.*, 1993).

GENETIC COUNSELING

The standing room only crowds at seminars hosted by NAMI hint at the desire—among family members and people with mental disorders—for more information about the genetics of mental disorders (Flynn, 1993). "[W]hat invariably happens is that people line up from the audience and they say, 'Let me tell you about my history. I have this, this, and that. What's the risk [to me and my family]?' " (Gershon, 1993). While genetic counseling for mental disorders apparently occurs rarely (Gottesman, 1991; U.S. Congress, 1992a)—an informal survey of genetic counselors in the New York area indicated that only a small number of people request counseling on mental illness (Marks, 1993)—consumer representatives at the OTA–NIMH workshop testified to a hunger for knowledge about genetics among people with mental disorders and their families (Beall, 1993).

> [T]here is a tremendous hunger for knowledge. Not for it to be packaged to us, but for us to be given both the uncertainty and the certainty. . . . Consumers want to know. The first thing that almost every consumer said [in a survey of 650 consumers in Virginia] is "I want to know, even if it's uncertain, even if it's complicated, I want to know," because mental illness for so many people has been presented as a mystery or as something that we are responsible for. To have information, even well-informed guesses given to us as that, is something we hunger for.

The relay of genetic information occurs formally in the context of genetic counseling. A recent report from the Institute of Medicine (1993) defines genetic counseling as:

> . . . the process by which individuals and families come to learn and understand relevant aspects of genetics; it is also the process for obtaining assistance in clarifying options available for their decisionmaking and coping with the significance of personal and family genetic knowledge in their lives.

The first question that needs to be addressed is whether genetic counseling is appropriate for mental disorders at all. A variety of factors would seem to answer no. The genetic contribution to these conditions is complex and incompletely understood. Certainly, there are no genetic tests for mental disorders. Even what is inherited is unclear. And genes by no means account for the whole picture. Mental disorders are generally considered multifactorial conditions; genetic and nongenetic factors are both involved. Furthermore, there is no known way to prevent the mental disorders considered in this report (although treatment may prevent relapse of symptoms in some conditions).

The enumerated rationale against genetic counseling for mental disorders neglects both the strengths and common application of genetic counseling as well as the desire for information among consumers. Genetic counseling is not simply about single gene disorders, disorders for which there are genetic tests, or the certain prediction of disease; it has a much broader application. The whole field of genetic counseling evolved around the concept of relaying risk information, probabilities, and uncertainties. Principles derived from genetic counseling—concerning risk communication and respect for client autonomy—can inform the relay of genetic information concerning mental disorders (Biesecker, 1993). As noted in a recently published psychiatric genetics text: "[A]n informed and responsible genetic counseling service has a small but definite current role, and this is likely to increase in the future" (McGuffin *et al.*, 1994).

It is true that no known interventions can prevent the development of the mental disorders discussed in this background paper. But, once again, mental disorders are not unique in this regard. Treatments effective for many people with mental disorders are available. Awareness of increased risk for a condition can help alert individuals to the earliest signs of a condition, permitting early treatment that may prevent the most debilitating symptoms and long-term impairment. Genetic counseling also offers an opportunity to correct common misperceptions about disorders with a genetic component: namely, that genetic conditions are impossible to treat or that these conditions require biological treatment (McGuffin *et al.*, 1994).

Many times a person with a severe mental disorder or his or her family members fear that children or siblings face a similar fate: a severely disabling and chronic condition. Not infrequently, severe mental disorders afflict generation after generation in a family. In this situation, information about the genetic risk for a condition can relieve fears. As noted at the workshop by the executive director of NAMI, and the mother of a daughter with schizophrenia (Flynn, 1993):

> Family members attending workshops and lectures on the genetics of mental illness almost always bring questions "This is my family. What do you think?" People's levels of anxiety are enormously high and almost always their reaction is "It's not as bad as I thought. We're not fated to have these dreadful illnesses in their most dreadful form just because we want to have a human experience and reproduce and have an extended family."

> So, there's an enormous amount of misunderstanding and partial understanding, even among families, and certainly families in the Alliance are as well educated

and knowledgeable about these disorders as any. So that the provision of knowledge offers an enormous amount of relief.

Recurrence risk is the most elementary information transmitted in
genetic counseling (Berg & Kirch, 1992; Biesecker, 1992; Institute of Medicine, 1993; Tsuang, 1978)—an individual's risk of inheriting a condition. For
mental disorders, no genetic test can lead to an individualized assessment.[2]
Rather, estimates of risk reflect pooled data from family studies, with
varying levels of information available for different disorders (Tables 1–3).
Empirical risk estimates convey the probability of mental disorder among
family members. For example, while approximately 1% of the general
population will develop schizophrenia, nearly 10% of those with a first-
degree relative with schizophrenia will become afflicted. First-degree relatives in general face a tenfold increased risk for schizophrenia.

Individuals with mental disorders and family members may find comfort in knowing that a mental disorder is not inevitable for loved ones. But
recurrence risk estimates do present difficulties. The concept of empirical
risk can be difficult to understand and act upon, which is why experts
in genetic counseling emphasize the importance of risk presentation and
interpretation (Bartels, LeRoy, & Caplan, 1993; Institute of Medicine, 1993;
U.S. Congress, 1992b). How an individual interprets risk estimates varies
depending on how the risk is perceived and communicated. Research into
several genetic conditions shows that a variety of factors influence the
perception of recurrence risk, including the nature of the illness and its
perceived burden. While little research has focused on the perception of
risk or perceived burden of mental disorders, existing data suggest diverging
experiences among primary and secondary consumers. In one small study,
92% of well family members versus 25% of affected individuals viewed
schizophrenia as a severe, debilitating disorder entailing extreme burden
(Schulz et al., 1982). Only 29% of the well family members, versus 66% of
individuals with schizophrenia, reported that they would have children. In
another study, 19 people with bipolar disorder and their well spouses were
asked about their perception of the disorder: approximately 50% of well
spouses compared with 5% of the bipolar patients indicated that they would
not have married and would not have had children if they had known more
about bipolar disorder (Targum et al., 1981).

Perceptions of risk and mental disorders are not the only obstacles
to genetic counseling. Simplified, recurrence risk data themselves can be
misleading. Recurrence risk estimates do not distinguish the severity of

[2]Even when genetic tests are available for a disorder, predictive ability can fall short of
the absolute, reflecting the specific genetic factors at play and always present possibilty of
human error.

Table 1
Averaged Risks of Mental Disorders[a]

	Schizophrenia	Bipolar disorder	Major depression	Obsessive-compulsive disorder	Panic disorder
General population	1.0%	0.8%	4.9%	2.6%	1.6%
First-degree relative (parent, child, or sibling)	9.0–13.0%[b]	4.0–9.0%	5.9–18.4%	25.0%	15.0–24.7%

[a]Source: Berg, K., & Kirch, D. G. (1992). National Institute of Mental Health, National Institutes of Health, U.S. Department of Health and Human Services, Bethesda.
[b]Risk is 46% when both parents are affected.

Table 2
Risk of Mood Disorder among Siblings of Individuals with a Major Mood Disorder by Status of Parents[a,b]

Study	Proband diagnosis	Sibling diagnosis	Risk to sibling when neither parent has a mood disorder (%)	Risk to sibling when at least one parent has a mood disorder (%)
Rudin, 1920	Mood disorder	Mood disorder	7.4	23.8
Schulz, 1930s	Mood disorder	Mood disorder	14.3	26.1
Luxenburger, 1930s	Mood disorder	Mood disorder	3.4	16.1
Pollock, Malzberg, & Fuller, 1939	Mood disorder	Mood disorder	1.3	3.8
Stendstedt, 1952	Mood disorder	Mood disorder	13.5	17.9
Reich, Clayton, & Winokus, 1969	Bipolar disorder	Mood disorder	10.0	21.0
Johnson & Leeman, 1977	Bipolar disorder	Mood disorder	18.4	23.2
Angst et al., 1980	Bipolar disorder	Bipolar disorder	1.2	5.6
	Bipolar disorder	Unipolar disorder	4.1	8.4

[a]Source: Tsuang, M. T., & Faraone, S. V. (1990). *The genetics of mood disorders.* Baltimore: Johns Hopkins University Press.
[b]Summary of data presented in Tsuang and Faraone (1990). Authors note in the text that empirical risks available on mood disorders generally do not take into account the multiple occurrence of such disorders in families. The exception is demonstrated in the table: the risk of mood disorders among siblings of individuals with these conditions when the status of the parents is known. All of the available studies indicate that the risk to a sibling is substantially increased if one of the parents is also ill.

Table 3
Familial Risk of Schizophrenia[a,b]

Relationship	Percentage of risk
General population	1
Spouses	2
Third-degree relatives	
First cousins	2
Second-degree relatives	
Uncles and aunts	2
Nephews and nieces	4
Grandchildren	5
Half siblings	6
First-degree relatives	
Parents	6
Siblings	9
Children	13
Siblings with one schizophrenic parent	17
Dizygotic twins	17
Monozygotic twins	48
Children with two parents with schizophrenia	46

[a]Source: Gottesman, I. I. (1991). *Schizophrenia genesis: The origins of madness*. San Francisco: Freeman.
[b]Risk estimates based on pooled data from the more than 40 systematic family and twin studies between 1920 and 1987.

disorder or the age of onset among family members. They provide no information about the genetic mechanisms at play. Recurrence risk in a particular family may greatly exceed or fall below the tabulated estimates. For example, if several members of a family have a particular mental disorder, usually with an early age of onset and severe course, other family members are more likely to develop the condition than average estimates of risk suggest.

Several implications flow from the limits on recurrence risk information for mental disorders. Sensitivity to varying understanding of illness and probability, as well as personal and cultural factors, must imbue genetic counseling. Average estimates of recurrence risk cannot stand alone; a careful diagnosis and family history provide an essential framework for the individualized interpretation of recurrence risk data. Finally, workshop participants concurred that more data are needed to better characterize specific risks that family members face in order to inform genetic counseling.

Genetic counseling extends beyond communicating recurrence risk. A complex tangle of concerns and questions impel the pursuit of information on genetics and mental disorders. One workshop participant, who is an expert in genetics and mental disorders, described a typical scenario (De-Paulo, 1993):

> A couple, who was contemplating having a family, sought genetic counseling on depression. The wife had experienced her first bout of severe depression. She expressed concern that symptoms may flair up postpartum, jeopardizing her job, the income from which was crucial for the family. They worried aloud about their relationship which was shaken by the depressive episode and the husband's ambivalence about having a child. These are common concerns expressed in genetic counseling: people are generally confronting a new diagnosis, fear the worst, not just in terms of risk to a child, but also in terms of the impact of the disorder on the family and the impact of a pregnancy and child-rearing on the health of a parent dealing with mental illness.

The panoply of concerns surrounding mental disorders and genetics underscores what genetic counselors increasingly realize; the relay of genetic information occurs in a therapeutic relationship (Bartels *et al.,* 1993; Biesecker, 1993; Institute of Medicine, 1993). Support, counseling, and follow-up services can assist individuals and their families in coping with a diagnosis of mental disorder, the risk family members face, and life decisions that may follow. Sensitivity to an individual's willingness and ability to receive genetic information is but the first demonstration of this psychotherapeutic component of genetic counseling. The provider of genetic services needs to be sensitive to the concept of the "teachable moment," the point at which an individual, couple, or family is most able to comprehend and absorb the information being given. A primary consumer at the OTA–NIMH workshop described the framework for the delivery of genetic information—the realization that one's life is altered by a mental disorder (Beall, 1993):

> I need to know that . . . the information is there if I need it. . . . As somebody with a primary psychiatric diagnosis, I will say that it is a process that one goes through of accepting that one first of all has an illness of this sort. I think that we go through stages that are almost like Kubler-Ross' stages of accepting death because who I believed I would be, who my family believed I would be, is not who I am. We die to ourselves. We die to our hopes, we die to our family's hopes and somehow we have to begin to find life beyond that. And we need to know that there is some information out there and we would like to draw from it because we also reconstruct our lives. We reconstruct who we are in the shifting ground of our disorder.

Providing information only on request is an overriding principle of genetic counseling. It signals not only a sensitivity to consumer receptivity, but also the value placed on individual autonomy in making life choices. Respect for individual autonomy drives nondirective counseling, which does not explicitly or implicitly make judgments on such personal decisions as marriage and childbearing. Medical geneticists harken to the wisdom of helping people at higher risk for a disorder to make decisions for themselves, by detailing the experiences and decisions that others have made (Conneally, 1993):

> Invariably I'm asked "Should I have children or not?" When that happens I tend to use Yogi Berra's edict. When you come to a fork in the road, take it. What I mean by that is that people confronting similar risks make different decisions and I provide them examples.
>
> One was Marjorie Guthrie. When she was invariably asked: Why did you have children, she would say, "Well, Woody had 45 fantastic years of life, very productive, etc., and I had three children. I am delighted I had them." That's one perspective.
>
> The other side is the case of the president of our Huntington's disease association; we had her come to talk to our medical students. She would say when asked that question: "Oh, I would never dream of bringing children into the world."
>
> I would point out both sides of these situations to this person and say "By the way, there are a lot of people on both sides and therefore whichever decision you're going to make, and I'm certainly not going to tell you which one to make, there are a lot of people who would agree with you" and leave it at that.

Many people with a mental disorder (or any condition that is genetic) and their family members confront the decision of whether that individual should have a child. Indeed, information on genetics is often sought in the context of family planning. In this context, highly charged issues can emerge for people with mental disorders (Flynn, 1993):

> When I talk to and listen to many consumers, they are not all nearly as supportive of this kind of effort as we might like them to be. The reason is because we have an unfortunate history in psychiatry, in public psychiatry in particular, of coercion, control, and sterilization in state hospitals. These things, we feel, have receded into the misty past but they're right up close to folks who are living with these disorders. So, when they hear you talking about genetic counseling, they think what you're really saying in code is, "I'm going to tell you how you should not have children. If I talk to you long enough and strong enough, you will believe me and you will do what I am counseling you to do."
>
> I certainly understand that's not what the goal of genetic counseling is, but that's how it's understood and that's how the public wants it to be done for people with these disorders. ... The outcome that many people are seeking is exactly the eugenic outcome that you described. ... That's what the whole incredibly powerful disability rights movement opposes. Mentally ill people are now part of that movement. The disability rights movement is not at all warm toward this aspect of your work because there's a very strong implicit statement about the value of their life as a disabled person. ... The way it's received by disabled people, and certainly I think that's the way many mentally ill people receive it, is that it's part of keeping them separate. It's part of saying, "You're not really normal. For instance, we don't think you should have a family life with children. ..."

> So, we have to be aware of what stigma in society has done, the high degree
> of defensiveness that it has created to the kind of information that we're trying
> to bring and the sense that many people have in the disability movement that
> there's a political undertone here of social control that is very, very worrisome.
> Having been so recently released from second-class status, having so recently
> seen themselves as full participants, they're very sensitive to anything that would
> seem to discount their value as whole people, real people, responsible people
> who can and should make judgments for themselves about their life.

The principle of nondirectiveness, so deeply embedded in genetic counseling, opposes the eugenic interventions that consumers fear. Psychiatric
geneticists generally spurn directive counseling against childbearing as well,
not only out of respect for consumer autonomy, but also on scientific
grounds (Gershon, 1990, 1993). "It needs to be said at the outset that there
is no place for public health campaigns persuading people with psychiatric
disorder or a strong family history of psychiatric disorder not to have
children" (McGuffin *et al.*, 1994). Recurrence risk for family members is
usually low for mental disorders (except when both parents are afflicted,
for example, with schizophrenia). These conditions are often treatable. And
the factors producing increased recurrence risk are not well understood.
Thus, the avoidance of childbearing is not scientifically supportable as a
means of primary prevention—eliminating mental disorders from the population.

While experts largely eschew eugenic principles and directive counseling on reproductive decisions for mental disorders, it would be dishonest
to ignore the difficult, indeed imperfect, translation of these principles into
practice. In the clinical realm, nondirective counseling, which does not
reveal the clinician's own view of the burden of illness or what's best for
the consumer, requires considerable skill (Bartels *et al.*, 1993; Biesecker,
1993; Murray, 1993). Society's negative view of mental disorders also
thwarts freedom of reproductive choice (Restinas, 1991; U.S. Congress,
1992b). Possible stigmatization can influence the reproductive decisions by
creating a sense of public disapproval (see next section). Secondarily, it
may result in depleted public resources and services for people with mental
disorders. Having a child with an increased risk of a mental disorder, when
services are inadequate for their care, is hardly an unhampered decision
(Nelkin, 1993).

Many experts take explicit exception to nondirective counseling of
people with a mental disorder when extremely disabled, raising questions
about decisionmaking and childrearing capabilities. For women with severe
mental disorders, childbearing presents several other issues, including birth
complications, potential teratogenic and other negative effects of some
psychotropic drugs on offspring, the effect of pregnancy and the postpartum

period on the mother's mental disorder, the mother's ability to handle the additional stress of raising a child, and the risk of adversely affecting the child's development. One workshop participant, a primary and secondary consumer, noted that all too often a mother with a severe mental disorder—in the midst of a symptom crisis—also faces the loss of custody of her children, a devastating reality that might be avoided with parental supports and adequate treatment (M. A. Beall, personal communication, July 21, 1994). In light of these concerns, a small body of research addresses issues around family planning for women with severe mental disorders (Coverdale *et al.*, 1993; Grunebaum *et al.*, 1971; McCullough *et al.*, 1994; Packer, 1992).

Workshop participants raised several other issues concerning genetic counseling and mental disorders: (1) the provision of genetic services, (2) multiple consumers of genetic counseling services, and (3) adoption and genetic counseling.

The Provision of Genetic Services

While genetic counselors and mental health care providers both have skills and expertise important for the relay of information on the genetics of mental disorders, professionals in neither field are fully trained to do so. Genetic counselors have knowledge of human genetics, are experienced in risk communication, and are steeped in a professional culture that respects individual autonomy. They typically do not have expertise in mental disorder diagnosis and treatment. Mental health care providers, on the other hand, offer expertise in the diagnosis and treatment of mental disorders; their knowledge of genetics and genetic counseling is limited. Given the dearth of genetic counselors—there are approximately 1500 genetic counselors in the United States, half of whom concentrate on prenatal counseling (Biesecker, 1993)—the most realistic solution to this knowledge gap is the transfer of competencies among professionals. Genetic counselors and experts in medical genetics can help educate mental health professionals about the relay of genetic information; also, they may increasingly form partnerships with mental health care providers.

Workshop participants noted another impediment to the delivery of genetic services: the way in which it is financed. Private insurance rarely reimburses genetic counseling as an independent service (Marks, 1993; Murray, 1993). Thus, most genetic counseling occurs in the context of a health care delivery team. Also, the reimbursement system is not geared to services that go to both an individual with a disorder and their families. Finally, any extension of genetic counseling to people with mental disorders will have to ensure that expertise reaches the public system of care, on which so many individuals with the most severe conditions rely.

Multiple Consumers of Genetic Counseling Services

The client or consumer of genetic counseling services includes not only an individual with a disorder, but also his or her family members and prospective spouses. All have an interest and may seek information on the inheritance of a condition. One workshop panelist noted the tensions that exist (Cox, 1993): "I don't have one client, I always have the family. So, I'm always juggling a lot of different balls in terms of who am I actually addressing, different issues for everybody in the family." Ideally, the provision of genetic information will not pit relatives, future spouses, and individuals with mental disorders against one another. In practice, however, information on diagnosis and the inheritance of mental disorders can lead to serious interpersonal conflict as well as raise legal and ethical concerns. In general, providers of genetic services try to balance their duties to maintain confidentiality—a primary but not absolute concern in the eyes of the law—against disclosing information, when confidentiality could cause harm to a third party (Andrews, 1991; Gottesman, 1993; Suter, 1993; see previous discussion).

Adoption and Genetic Counseling

It is not uncommon for women with severe psychiatric disorder to give up their children for adoption. Prospective parents therefore may have an interest in learning the risk for serious mental disorder in their adopted offspring. One workshop panelist indicated that "probably the most frequent call I get is from a prospective adoptive parent who goes through regular adoption agencies in the United States and finds out that the child has a mother with schizophrenia (DeLisi, 1993). Adoptive parents face barriers to information. In addition to the limited number of professionals able to give genetic information on mental disorders, access to information on the mental history of biological parents may be lacking (Blair, 1992).

PUBLIC PERCEPTIONS AND SOCIAL IMPLICATIONS

Research does not move forward in a social vacuum, simply unveiling new knowledge. Obviously, biomedical research has as one primary goal the improvement of clinical care. But the interface between research and society goes beyond clinical practice. Scientific advances become the tools of public opinion and social policy (Nelkin & Tancredi, 1994). Conversely, the social perception of a scientific approach can fuel popular support—or opposition. The subject of the workshop—genetics and mental disorders—invokes powerful images and arouses intense public reactions. This section considers public perceptions of genetics and mental disorders, how they intermingle, and some of the social and public policy issues that emerge.

Molecular genetics has become a modern-day celebrity (Nelkin, 1992; Nelkin & Lindee, 1995). Featured on the front pages of newspapers and popular magazines, molecular genetics is often described as instruction manual, crystal ball, and pharmacopoeia all rolled up into one (for a recent example, see Elmer-Dewitt, 1994). This air of expectation that surrounds genetic research has led many commentators to express the hope that human diseases will be vanquished and even many social ills will be eliminated (Cook-Deegan, 1994; Keller, 1992; Maddox, 1993). The general public apparently accepts this expectation, with national surveys showing enthusiasm for genetic testing and gene therapy (March of Dimes Birth Defects Foundation, 1992).

Some analysts worry about the hyperbole and value-laden symbols used to describe molecular genetics. Genes are characterized as good or bad; there are popular references to people "going shopping" for genes when choosing a mate or adopting a child; complex traits and behavior are boiled down to DNA fragments. Many liken genetics with invariable or unchangeable characteristics. In an analysis of "The Social Power of Genetic Information," one workshop participant characterized how gene-talk has infiltrated the public's psyche (Nelkin, 1992).

> You can be sure that genetic ideas have been popularized when you see a button saying "Gene Police! You—Out of the Pool"; or a Mother's Day card, to a daughter who is herself a mother, that says on the front, "What a good Mother you are," and on the inside, "It's all in the genes." Even the advertising industry seems to have assimilated genetic concepts: an ad for a BMW boasts its "genetic advantage."

Slogans by themselves are hardly dangerous. But their influence on public attitude may be, especially among people unfamiliar with genetic principles—as is the norm (U.S. Department of Energy, 1992). Perhaps most ironically, expressed genetic "triumphalism," as the editor of the prestigious journal *Nature* termed it (Maddox, 1993), fuels a backlash against the very science it once celebrated. A recent article in *Time* magazine noted that "[t]here is already talk of a genetic backlash, a revolt against the notion that we are our genes, or as one critic put it, 'that our Genes R Us' " (Elmer-Dewitt, 1994). Data from surveys also convey public fears and concerns about genetic testing and genetic engineering (Elmer-Dewitt, 1994; March of Dimes Birth Defects Foundation, 1992). Researchers of the genetics of mental disorders, who participated in the OTA–NIMH workshop, described how just a few years transformed them from scientific heroes to pariahs among their peers (DeLisi, 1993). In a recent manuscript, a scientist who participated in the workshop notes that genetics is often equated with Nazism. "Critics of this enterprise are quick to associate contemporary strategies with the lurid and disquieting past abuses of biology by the Nazis, resulting in the sterilization or murder of thousands of mental patients, the physically handicapped, and millions of 'non-Aryans' during the Holocaust" (Gottesman, 1994). Similarly, a researcher studying twins who are discordant for schizophrenia notes in a recent text that he was "publicly called 'a new Mengele' by a psychiatrist at a national conference" (Torrey *et al.*, 1994). He concludes that "[f]or a few people it seems that anybody who studies twins is automatically assumed to be a fascist or worse" (Torrey, *et al.*, 1994).

Withered support for research is not the only worrisome result of exaggerated or simpleminded claims about genetics. The public's perception of genetics is a primary thread in the fabric of public policy. Many analysts express alarm at the potential discriminatory use of genetic information, falsely perceived as forecasting a certain, unyielding, or completely incapacitating fate (Allen & Ostrer, 1993; Natowicz, Alper, & Alper, 1992). A preliminary case study describes some of the discriminatory consequences of such viewpoints (Billings *et al.*, 1992):

> Genetic conditions are regarded by many social institutions as extremely serious, disabling, or even lethal conditions without regard to the fact that many individuals with "abnormal" genotypes will either be perfectly healthy, have medical conditions which can be controlled by treatment, or experience only mild forms of a disease. As a result of this misconception, decisions by such institutions as insurance companies and employers are made solely on the basis of an associated diagnostic label rather than on the actual health status of the individual or family.... Once labeled ... an individual may suffer serious consequences.... These include inability to get a job, health insurance, or life insurance, being unable to change jobs or move to a different state because of the possibility of losing insurance, and not being allowed to adopt a child.

Genetic discrimination has received considerable attention from policymakers and analysts. In fact, 5% of the National Institutes of Health's National Center for Human Genome Research budget—$5 million in fiscal year 1992—is devoted to the task of addressing the Ethical, Legal, and Social Implications (ELSI) of genetic information. Among the most discussed issues are insurance and employment discrimination on the basis of genetic test results.

While genetic information and the perception of genetics may serve to limit access to health care, its social influence may be more insidious. Public pressure may mount against individuals viewed as passing on disease genes to their offspring. Citing survey results, a recent OTA report concluded that "stigmatization of carriers [of the gene for cystic fibrosis] is likely to focus on beliefs that it is irresponsible and immoral for people who could transmit disability to their children to reproduce" (U.S. Congress, 1992b). In response to a 1990 general population survey, 39% said "every woman who is pregnant should be tested to determine if the baby has any serious genetic defect." Nearly 10% of those surveyed expressed the belief that a woman should be required by law to have an abortion rather than have the government help pay for the child's care. Public opinion may even turn against bringing a child into the world with a benign genetic condition. The public response to TV anchorwoman Bree Walker Lampley's pregnancy is illustrative. When she became pregnant with her second child, she found herself the focus of Los Angeles radio talk show attacks. Ms. Lampley has a genetic condition—ectrodactyly—which manifests as the absence of one or more fingers or toes. Because her offspring are at a 50% risk of inheriting the condition, the radio talk show callers and host criticized Lampley's pregnancy.

Mental disorders are among the most stigmatized of health conditions. Although attitudes toward mental disorders appear to be improving (Clements, 1993; F. D. Burgmann, personal communication, July 30, 1994), data continue to show that the public is uneducated about mental disorders, fearful of them, and hostile to people with these conditions (U.S. Congress, 1992a, 1994). For example, a recent national survey of public attitudes toward people with disabilities shows that from the public's perspective, mental disorders are the most disturbing of all disabling conditions (National Organization on Disability, 1991). Many individuals harbor beliefs that bad parenting, personal inadequacy, weakness of character, or sinfulness lie at the root of severe mental disorders (U.S. Congress, 1992a). The news and entertainment media promote these stigmatizing views with their routine presentation of people with mental disorders as incompetent, ineffectual, and violent (U.S. Congress, 1992a, 1994).

Ignorance and negative attitudes, combined with other factors, wreak havoc on the lives of people with mental disorders. Data from surveys and other research show the tragic consequences: people with severe mental disorders suffer poor self-esteem and discrimination in employment, housing, and access to health care (Link, 1987; U.S. Congress, 1994).

The negative attitudes attached to mental disorders aggrieve family members as well. In addition to becoming the most significant care-provider, family members suffer psychological consequences.

Subjective burden—the family's distress over the pain and altered life prospects of their mentally ill relative—is exacerbated by these stigmatizing events. Reactions to perceived social censure become intertwined with responses to the sorrows and demands of the illness itself. Emotional reactions to major mental illness in a family member frequently include bewilderment, fear, denial, self-blame, sorrow, grieving, and empathic suffering. The added perception of stigma may elicit rage and resentment or intensify depression and social withdrawal. [Lefley, 1992]

It is on this stage of stigmatization and discrimination that the social influence of genetic models of mental disorders will play out. What is or will be the result of the comingling of public perceptions of genetics and mental disorders? Although few research data address this issue, workshop participants and other commentators describe the complex blend of views. On an undercurrent of fear, many primary and secondary consumers express relief and optimism concerning genetic research of mental disorders.

I think it's a complex issue but if you look at the kind of stigma that is most painful to people who have chronic psychiatric disabilities, discovering the scientific substrate and the underpinnings of these disorders has been profoundly destigmatizing, I would say, in the last decade. And I think it will continue to function that way. [Beall, 1993]

Clinicians echo this perception as the words of Dr. Raymond DePaulo (1993) reveal:

Families ... do express fears. But I think, by and large, they're greatly relieved right now that we're seriously going at this enterprise. And they take hope, not just from the fact that Freud was wrong and it isn't mother's fault, but even more from the fact that people are seriously working on finding the causes of these disorders.

Many people with mental disorders and their families look forward to the results of genetic research, because it offers promise of improved understanding of their condition and hope for improved treatment (Wahl & Harman, 1989). The very image of mental disorders as biological—genetic—is viewed as destigmatizing, thus offering comfort for some. "Proliferation of biogenetic research findings ... has somewhat softened the older prejudices against families" (Lefley, 1992).

A note of caution was sounded at the OTA–NIMH workshop, in terms of the potential discriminatory consequences of genetic data and the backlash against research described above (Billings, 1993):

I think that it's quite right that in general ... families affected with mental disorders have a great belief in the value of research ... [that it will] change their status for the better. And I think that's a realistic and hopeful and good thing. I think that it must be tempered, however, by a realistic appraisal of the immediate impacts of that research. For instance, the results of research becoming diagnostic tools can have an immediate negative impact on them, let's say with employers or insurers or whatever, using the information in a discriminatory way. The other thing I would say is that . . . I think that there's an issue of how research gets transmitted to the public as well. You know, I see a lot of people who are in cystic fibrosis groups or whatever, who are disillusioned at some level with research, with genetic research. It's clearly true in mental disorders as well . . . I think that there has to be, within the research community, some recognition that crummy linkage studies have an impact and it's not always so good.

Recognizing the destigmatizing influences of genetic research, one workshop participant evoked the lessons of history in his note of caution (Cook-Deegan, 1993):

> There's a two-edged sword here. One of the roles of genetics in the 1980s has been to use genetics as a destigmatizing force. That is, the ability to say that there are genes involved in a disorder proves that it is more like heart disease or cancer because it's a physical disorder. There's something broken in your brain. In essence, it's an assault on the Freudian determinism of parenting causing schizophrenia. That's very powerful. But at the same time, we've got a carryover of genetic determinism from the past where, after all, in Germany, it was the folks with psychiatric disorders who were believed to have the disorders for genetic reasons who were the first victims of eugenics. . . . So . . . we've got a very strange mix of cross currents going on here. We've got one social current that says "We need genetics to de-stigmatize" but we seem to have forgotten the history that suggests that genetics can be used as a label effect—once that label is imposed, it sticks and can be used against the individual and family.

History teaches us that science and prejudice can combine in ways ruinous to people with stigmatized conditions and their families. The history of screening for sickle-cell anemia in this country provides an example (U.S. Congress, 1992b). Sickle-cell anemia impairs red blood cell flow through the circulatory system, causing complications in organ systems throughout the body. This painful, incurable, and sometimes fatal genetic condition has a high incidence among African-Americans, with 1 in 400 newborns having sickle-cell anemia. One in ten or eleven have the sickle-cell trait. Individuals with the sickle-cell trait have a normal and healthy life but if they marry another carrier can have a child with sickle-cell disease. A massive screening program for sickle-cell trait was undertaken in the 1970s, so that couples could be informed of their risks of having affected children. While at first glance, screening programs offered an inexpensive benefit to African-American citizens—indeed, most laws were drafted and promoted by African-American legislators at the height of the civil rights movement—early programs suffered from misinformation and discrimination against carriers. Some state statutes consistently contained blatant medical and scientific errors. Almost every state law failed to insist on using the most sensitive assay available. Controversy also focused on the racial distribution of sickle-cell mutations and the target screening population. The laws were seen by many citizens as racist eugenic measures aimed at reducing the number of marriages between carriers and decreasing the number of pregnancies at risk for affected children of a minority population. The fact that the programs were largely designed and operated by Caucasians fueled fears of genocide. Most state laws failed to provide adequate education and counseling for persons with sickle-cell anemia or the trait. Those diagnosed with sickle-cell trait were often told they should not have children, that childbirth would be hazardous, or other untruths. State laws also failed to provide public education to guard against discrimination and stigmatization. Stories of job and insurance discrimination multiplied as screening programs proliferated. Other screening programs have had similar consequences for the insurability and employability of those identified as predisposed to genetic conditions (Nelkin & Tancredi, 1994).

The eugenics movement earlier this century offers an even more terrifying example of the potentially dangerous mix between genetics and prejudice against mental disorders. In Nazi Germany and the United States, people with mental disorders were among the initial targets of eugenic policies (Duster, 1990; Garver & Garver, 1991; Gottesman, 1993; Meyer, 1988). A number of scientific discoveries planted the seeds of eugenic policies in the 19th and 20th centuries. Sir Francis Galton, a cousin of Darwin who coined the term *eugenics,* observed that many accomplished men of his day were linked by bloodlines, which led to his belief that proper matings could produce a race with enhanced intellectual, behavioral, and physical characteristics—positive eugenics. In addition, Galton and others developed statistical techniques that permitted the quantitative analysis of inherited traits. Social, political, and economic factors fertilized the growth of the eugenics movement. National attention was increasingly focused on social issues of unemployment, criminality, prostitution, and chronic alcoholism. Also, concerns arose that increased immigration from southern and eastern Europe was drawing the United States away from its "Anglo-Saxon superiority."

Public policies executed these scientific and social developments. At the federal level, eugenic policies took the form of increasingly restrictive immigration laws. Eugenicists, asserting the simple inheritance of such traits as lunacy, epilepsy, alcoholism, pauperism, criminality, and feeblemindedness, proffered scientific rationales for excluding individuals from entry to the United States. While authentic advances in genetics seeded the eugenics movement, they provided no evidence for the simple inheritance of the traits mentioned above. Eugenic considerations also prompted states to enact laws regarding compulsory sterilization. In 1907, Indiana passed the first law legalizing the compulsory sterilization of inmates at the state reformatory. By 1931, 30 states had passed compulsory sterilization laws applying to individuals categorized as feebleminded, alcoholic, epileptic, sexually deviant, or mentally ill. Individuals with mental disorders made up half of the 64,000 persons in this country sterilized for eugenic reasons between 1907 and 1964. When eugenic sterilization laws were challenged in 1927, the U.S. Supreme Court ruled the practice constitutional.

Many consider that the current application of immigration and compulsory sterilization laws suggests that eugenics is no longer a major concern. Furthermore, the understanding that mental disorders do not have a simple genetic basis and that nongenetic factors play an important role would seem to limit the potential of eugenic policies. Perhaps most important, American repulsion by the Nazi legacy and the emphasis in this country on individual reproductive rights also make state-determined eugenic policies unlikely. But, as noted above, indirect pressure not to have children may well come to bear on individuals seen to have a greater genetic risk of mental disorders; society may brand them irresponsible or immoral for transmitting disorders to their children. And eugenic policies may lurk abroad. In China, a draft law on "eugenics and health protection" presented to the Eighth National People's Congress (NPC) in 1993, proposed that people with diseases such as mental illness "which can be passed on through birth" be banned from marrying (Dickson, 1994).

SUMMARY AND CONCLUSIONS

People with mental disorders and their families participate in research, benefit from its results, and feel the impact of its social dissemination. Workshop participants discussed these clinical and social implications of research into the genetics of mental disorders. At least three issues stand at the fore of any attempt to bridge the gap between research and society: family involvement, the nature of mental disorders, and the need for education.

Historically, ethical guidelines and public policy largely have focused on the well-being of the individual, as research participant, consumer of clinical services, and member of society. Genetic research broadens this approach, extending the circle of concern to family members in addition to the afflicted individual. Family members are necessary participants in research raising issues around consent and confidentiality. Family members often seek information on genetic status, which raises potential conflicts. Any social effect of genetic research—for example, its use to limit access to health care—will obtrude on individuals with mental disorders and family members alike. While workshop participants recognized the potential clash of interests between family members and affected individuals, many expressed the belief that a framework of benevolence could lead to relevant guidance for research, clinical practice, and public policy—developments that are sorely needed.

Two features of mental disorders color genetic research and its translation into practice and policy. First, mental disorders can sometimes circumscribe an individual's decisionmaking ability. The impact of some mental disorder symptoms raises issues around informed consent for research participation and informed clinical decisionmaking. Advocating the importance of individual autonomy, workshop panelists strongly asserted the need to take seriously and perhaps foster further guidelines and policies that increase the meaningful participation of people with mental disorders in research and clinical care, so as to better protect their rights and well-being.

The second feature of mental disorders that permeates genetic research is the stigma attached to these conditions. The ignorance and negative attitudes attached to mental disorders encumber research and clinical care, heightening concerns about confidentiality. The stigma also drives support for this research among many consumers, and, paradoxically, could fuel its abusive application. This social reality animates the final issue put forth by workshop participants: the need for education.

Educational needs extend to several spheres. Researchers and individuals participating in the review of research need information about the clinical and ethical issues raised by research into the genetics of mental disorders. Mental health care providers need information about the genetics of mental disorders and the practice of delivering such information to requesting consumers. Similarly, genetic counselors need information on the nature, diagnosis, and treatment of mental disorders. Finally, society at large needs information about the nature of genetics and mental disorders, in order to diminish fears and stigmatization and to help inoculate against discriminatory policies.

REFERENCES

Allen, W., & Ostrer, H. (1993). Anticipating unfair uses of genetic information. *American Journal of Human Genetics, 53*, 16–21.

Andrews, L. B. (1991). Legal aspects of genetic information. *The Yale Journal of Biology and Medicine, 64*, 29–40.

Bartels, D. M., LeRoy, B. S., & Caplan, A. L. (Eds.). (1993). *Prescribing our future: Ethical challenges in genetic counseling.* Berlin: Aldine de Gruyter.

Beall, M. A. (1993). Vice President, Virginia Alliance for the Mentally Ill, and Chair, Virginia Mental Health Consumers' Association, Richmond, VA, remarks at "Understanding the Role of Genetic Factors in Mental Illness: Bridging the Gap Between Research and

Society," a workshop sponsored by the Office of Technology Assessment and the National Institute of Mental Health, Washington, DC, January 21–22, 1993.

Berg, K., & Kirch, D. G. (1992). National Institute of Mental Health, National Institutes of Health, *Genetic counseling in psychiatry,* draft.

Biesecker, B. B. (1993). Genetic Counselor, National Center for Human Genome Research, National Institutes of Health, Bethesda, MD, remarks at "Understanding the Role of Genetic Factors in Mental Illness: Bridging the Gap Between Research and Society," a workshop sponsored by the Office of Technology Assessment and the National Institute of Mental Health, Washington, DC, January 21–22, 1993.

Billings, P. R. (1993). Chief Medical Officer, Department of Veterans' Affairs Medical Center, Palo Alto, CA, remarks at "Understanding the Role of Genetic Factors in Mental Illness: Bridging the Gap Between Research and Society," a workshop sponsored by the Office of Technology Assessment and the National Institute of Mental Health, Washington, DC, January 21–22, 1993.

Billings, P. R., Kohn, M. A., de Cuevas, M., *et al.* (1992). Discrimination as a consequence of genetic testing. *American Journal of Human Genetics, 50,* 476–482.

Blair, D. M. B. (1992). Lifting the genealogical veil: A blueprint for legislative reform of the disclosure of health-related information in adoption. *North Carolina Law Review, 70,* 681–779.

Clements, M. (1993, October 31). What we say about mental illness. *Parade Magazine,* pp. 4–6.

Conneally, P. M. (1993). Distinguished Professor of Medical Genetics and Neurology, Indiana University School of Medicine, Indianapolis, remarks at "Understanding the Role of Genetic Factors in Mental Illness: Bridging the Gap Between Research and Society," a workshop sponsored by the Office of Technology Assessment and the National Institute of Mental Health, Washington, DC, January 21–22, 1993.

Cook-Deegan, R. M. (1993). Director, Division of Bio-Behavioral Sciences and Mental Disorders, Institute of Medicine, Washington, DC, remarks at "Understanding the Role of Genetic Factors in Mental Illness: Bridging the Gap Between Research and Society," a workshop sponsored by the Office of Technology Assessment and the National Institute of Mental Health, Washington, DC, January 21–22, 1993.

Cook-Deegan, R. M. (1994). *The gene wars: Science, politics, and the human genome.* New York: Norton.

Coverdale, J. H., Bayer, T. L., McCullough, L. B., *et al.* (1993). Respecting the autonomy of chronically mentally ill women in decisions about contraception. *Hospital and Community Psychiatry, 44,* 671–674.

Cox, D. R. (1993). Professor, School of Medicine, Stanford University, Palo Alto, CA, remarks at "Understanding the Role of Genetic Factors in Mental Illness: Bridging the Gap Between Research and Society," a workshop sponsored by the Office of Technology Assessment and the National Institute of Mental Health, Washington, DC, January 21–22, 1993.

DeLisi, L. E. (1993). Professor of Psychiatry, Research Foundation SUNY, remarks at "Understanding the Role of Genetic Factors in Mental Illness: Bridging the Gap Between Research and Society," a workshop sponsored by the Office of Technology Assessment and the National Institute of Mental Health, Washington, DC, January 21–22, 1993.

DePaulo, J. R. (1993). Associate Professor, Johns Hopkins University, School of Medicine, Baltimore, remarks at "Understanding the Role of Genetic Factors in Mental Illness: Bridging the Gap Between Research and Society," a workshop sponsored by the Office of Technology Assessment and the National Institute of Mental Health, Washington, DC, January 21–22, 1993.

186   LAURA LEE HALL

Dickson, D. (1994). Concerns grow over China's plans to reduce number of 'inferior births.' *Nature, 367,* 3.

Duster, T. (1990). *Backdoor to eugenics.* New York: Routledge.

Elmer-Dewitt, P. (1994, January 17). The genetic revolution. *Time,* pp. 46–53.

Flynn, L. (1993). Executive Director, National Alliance for the Mentally Ill, Arlington, VA, remarks at "Understanding the Role of Genetic Factors in Mental Illness: Bridging the Gap Between Research and Society," a workshop sponsored by the Office of Technology Assessment and the National Institute of Mental Health, Washington, DC, January 21–22, 1993.

Frankel, M. S., & Teich, A. H. (Eds.). (1993). *The genetic frontier: Ethics, law, and policy.* Washington, DC: American Association for the Advancement of Science.

Garver, K. L., & Garver, B. (1991). Eugenics: Past, present, and future. *American Journal of Human Genetics, 49,* 1109–1118.

Gershon, E. S. (1990). Genetics. In F. K. Goodwin & K. R. Jamison (Eds.), *Manic-depressive illness.* London: Oxford University Press.

Gerhson, E. (1993). Chief, Clinical Neurogenetics Branch, National Institute of Mental Health, National Institutes of Health, Bethesda, remarks at "Understanding the Role of Genetic Factors in Mental Illness: Bridging the Gap Between Research and Society," a workshop sponsored by the Office of Technology Assessment and the National Institute of Mental Health, Washington, DC, January 21–22, 1993.

Gottesman, I. I. (1991). *Schizophrenia genesis: The origins of madness.* San Francisco: Freeman.

Gottesman, I. I. (1993). Professor, University of Virginia, Charlottesville, remarks at "Understanding the Role of Genetic Factors in Mental Illness: Bridging the Gap Between Research and Society," a workshop sponsored by the Office of Technology Assessment and the National Institute of Mental Health, Washington, DC, January 21–22, 1993.

Gottesman, I. I. (1994). Schizophrenia epigenesis: Past, present, and future. *Acta Psychiatrica Scandinavica, 90*(Suppl. 384, 26–33.

Grisso, T., & Appelbaum, P. S. (1991). Mentally ill and non-mentally-ill patients' abilities to understand informed consent disclosures for medication. *Law and Human Behavior, 15,* 377–388.

Grunebaum, H. U., Abernethy, V. D., Rofman, E. S., et al. (1971). The family planning attitudes, practices, and motivations of mental patients. *American Journal of Psychiatry, 128,* 740–744.

Honberg, R. (1993). Legal Advocate, National Alliance for the Mentally Ill, Arlington, VA, remarks at "Understanding the Role of Genetic Factors in Mental Illness: Bridging the Gap Between Research and Society," a workshop sponsored by the Office of Technology Assessment and the National Institute of Mental Health, Washington, DC, January 21–22, 1993.

Institute of Medicine. (1993). *Assessing genetic risks: Implications for health social policy.* Washington, DC: National Academy Press.

Jamison, K. R. (1993). *Touched with fire.* New York: Free Press.

Keller, E. F. (1992). Nature, nurture, and the Human Genome Project. In D. J. Kevles & L. Hood (Eds.), *The code of codes: Scientific and social issues in the Human Genome Project.* Cambridge, MA: Harvard University Press.

Lefley, H. P. (1992). The stigmatized family. In P. J. Fink & A. Tasman (Eds.), *Stigma and mental illness.* Washington, DC: American Psychiatric Press.

Link, B. G. (1987). Understanding labeling effects in the area of mental disorders: An assessment of the effects of expectations of rejection. *American Sociological Review, 52,* 96–112.

McCullough, L. B., Coverdale, J., Bayer, T., et al. (1992). Ethically justified guidelines for family planning interventions to prevent pregnancy in female patients with chronic mental illness. *American Journal of Obstetrics and Gynecology, 167,* 19–25.

McGuffin, P., Owen, M. J., O'Donovan, M. C., *et al.* (1994). *Seminars in psychiatric genetics.* London: Gaskell.

Maddox, J. (1993). Willful public misunderstanding of genetics. *Nature, 364,* 281.

March of Dimes Birth Defects Foundation. (1992, September). *Genetic testing and gene therapy: National survey findings.* Washington, DC.

Marks, J. H. (1993). Director, Human Genetics Program, Sarah Lawrence College, Bronxville, NY, remarks at "Understanding the Role of Genetic Factors in Mental Illness: Bridging the Gap Between Research and Society, a workshop sponsored by the Office of Technology Assessment and the National Institute of Mental Health, Washington, DC, January 21–22, 1993.

Meyer, J.-E. (1988). The fate of the mentally ill in Germany during the Third Reich. *Psychological Medicine, 18,* 575–581.

Murray, R. J., Jr. (1993). Professor, Howard University College of Medicine, Washington, DC, remarks at "Understanding the Role of Genetic Factors in Mental Illness: Bridging the Gap Between Research and Society," a workshop sponsored by the Office of Technology Assessment and the National Institute of Mental Health, Washington, DC, January 21–22, 1993.

National Organization on Disability. (1991). Public attitudes toward people with disabilities," survey conducted by Louis Harris and Associates, Inc. Washington, DC.

Natowicz, M. R., Alper, J. K., & Alper, J. S. (1992). *Genetic discrimination and the law. American Journal of Human Genetics, 50,* 465–475.

Nelkin, D. (1992). The social power of genetic information. In D. J. Kevles & L. Hood (Eds.), *The code of codes: Scientific and social issues in the Human Genome Project.* Cambridge, MA: Harvard University Press.

Nelkin, D. (1993). Professor, New York University, New York, remarks at "Understanding the Role of Genetic Factors in Mental Illness: Bridging the Gap Between Research and Society," a workshop sponsored by the Office of Technology Assessment and the National Institute of Mental Health, Washington, DC, January 21–22, 1993.

Nelkin, D., & Lindee, S. (1995). *The DNA mystique: The gene as a cultural icon.* New York: Freeman.

Nelkin, D., & Tancredi, L., (1994). *Dangerous diagnostics: The social power of biological information* (2nd ed). (Chicago: University of Chicago Press.

Packer, S. (1992). Family planning for women with bipolar disorder. *Hospital and Community Psychiatry, 43,* 479–481.

Restinas, J. (1991). The impact of prenatal technology upon attitudes toward disabled infants. *Research in the Sociology of Health Care, 9,* 75–102.

Schulz, P. M., Schulz, S. C., Dibble, E., *et al.* (1982). Patient and family attitudes about schizophrenia: Implications for genetic counseling. *Schizophrenia Bulletin, 8,* 504–513.

Shore, D. (1993). Director, Schizophrenia Research Branch, National Institute of Mental Health, National Institutes of Health, Rockville, MD, remarks at "Understanding the Role of Genetic Factors in Mental Illness: Bridging the Gap Between Research and Society," a workshop sponsored by the Office of Technology Assessment and the National Institute of Mental Health, Washington, DC, January 21–22, 1993.

Shore, D., Berg, K., Wynne, D., *et al.* (1993). Legal and ethical issues in psychiatric genetic research. *American Journal of Medical Genetics (Neuropsychiatric Genetics), 48,* 17–21.

Suter, S. M. (1993). Whose genes are these anyway?: Familial conflicts over access to genetic information. *Michigan Law Review, 91,* 1854–1908.

Targum, S. D., Dibble, E. D., Davenport, Y. B., *et al.* (1981). The Family Attitudes Question-naire: Patients' and spouses' views of bipolar illness. *Archives of General Psychiatry, 38,* 562–568.

Torrey, E. F., Bowler, A. E., Taylor, E. H., *et al.* (1994). *Schizophrenia and manic-depressive disorder: The biological roots of mental illness as revealed by the landmark study of identical twins.* New York: Basic Books.

Tsuang, M. T. (1978). Genetic counseling for psychiatric patients and their families. *American Journal of Psychiatry, 135,* 1465–1475.

Tsuang, M. T., & Faraone, S. V. (1990). The genetics of mood disorders Baltimore: Johns Hopkins University Press.

U.S. Congress, Office of Technology Assessment. (1992a). *The biology of mental disorders* (OTA-BA-538). Washington, DC: U.S. Government Printing Office.

U.S. Congress, Office of Technology Assessment. (1992b). *Cystic fibrosis and DNA tests: Implications of carrier screening* (OTA-BA-532). Washington, DC: U.S. Government Printing Office.

U.S. Congress, Office of Technology Assessment. (1993). *Biomedical ethics in U.S. public policy—Background paper* (OTA-BP-BBS-105). Washington, DC: U.S. Government Printing Office.

U.S. Congress, Office of Technology Assessment. (1994). *Psychiatric disabilities, employment, and the Americans With Disabilities Act* (OTA-BP-BBS-124). Washington, DC: U.S. Government Printing Office.

U.S. Department of Energy, Los Alamos Science. (1992). *The Human Genome Project* No. 20.

U.S. Department of Health and Human Services, National Institutes of Health, Office for the Protection from Research Risk. (1993). *Human genetic research.*

U.S. Department of Health, Education, and Welfare, National Commission for the Protection of Human Subjects of Biomedical and Behavioral Research. (1978). *The Belmont Report: Ethical principles and guidelines for the protection of human subjects of research.* Washington, DC: U.S. Government Printing Office.

Wahl, O. F., & Harman, C. R. (1989). Family views of stigma. *Schizophrenia Bulletin, 15,* 131–139.

CHAPTER 9

Bioethics and the Federal Government
Some Implications for Psychiatric Genetics

ROBERT MULLAN COOK-DEEGAN

> Identify the requirements for informed consent to participation in biomedical
> and behavioral research . . . by the institutionalized mentally infirm . . . to deter-
> mine the nature of the consent obtained from such persons or their legal represen-
> tatives before such persons were involved in such research; the adequacy of the
> information given them respecting the nature and purpose of the research,
> procedures to be used, risks and discomforts, anticipated benefits from the
> research, and other matters necessary for informed consent; and the competence
> and the freedom of the persons to make a choice for or against involvement in
> such research. [National Commission, 1978d]

Psychiatric genetics lies at the confluence of several turbulent streams in
social policy. It increasingly involves the tools of molecular genetics, one
of the fastest evolving areas of modern science; it taps into the ethics of
genetic research, particularly the special aspects of family studies; and
it deals with clinical conditions that by definition hinder normal mental
functions, thus complicating the process by which individuals agree to participate in research. The symptoms of psychiatric conditions are behavioral,
and the study of how genes influence behavior has long been attended by
controversy. As historian Daniel Kevles noted, "In its ongoing fascination
with questions of behavior, human genetics will undoubtedly yield informa-

ROBERT MULLAN COOK-DEEGAN • National Academy of Sciences, Washington, D.C.
20418.

Genetics and Mental Illness: Evolving Issues for Research and Society, edited by Laura Lee
Hall. Plenum Press, New York, 1996.

tion that may be wrong, or socially volatile, or, if the history of eugenic science is any guide, both" (Kevles & Hood, 1992).

Federal policies pertain directly to several aspects of psychiatric genetics. Most basic biomedical research, including psychiatric genetics, is funded by the National Institutes of Health, a federal agency. The regulations governing the involvement of human subjects in research are set at the federal level, and the federal Office of Protection from Research Risks is responsible for monitoring compliance with them. Federal bioethics commissions have played an important role in addressing not only issues of involving human subjects in research, but also in dealing publicly with a broader array of issues. This chapter reviews these aspects of federal policy by looking first at some distinctive aspects of psychiatric research, then at the emergence of a research program to address social, legal, and ethical issues connected to the Human Genome Project, and finally turning to the nation's experience with federal bioethics commissions. A concluding section looks at how a combination of empirical studies and a bioethics commission can contribute to clarifying federal policy choices.

Bioethics is a loosely defined, interdisciplinary field that concerns itself explicitly with answering the question "what is the right thing to do?" Deciding what is right must usually be done in the face of considerable uncertainty. Psychiatric genetic research confronts several types of uncertainty. Some derives from ignorance about the underlying biology of the disorders themselves. This is, for the most part, a problem for science. Some comes from an incomplete set of facts that pertain to any specific decision, from an incomplete story. This can only be dealt with by processes for gathering facts that pertain to a particular case. And some results from lack of clarity about what is morally right, and this is the domain of bioethics. Bioethics must begin with solid science and good facts, but it does not end there. Bioethics proceeds from a base of the best available information to consider actions that fall within the boundaries of what is morally acceptable. The signature of bioethics is an explicit analysis of what ought to be, following a description of what is.

In public policy regarding biomedical research, bioethics has been quite useful in defining the criteria that should be used in formulating federal rules. Rules governing the participation of human subjects in research, about definitions of death, about how health care decisions are made and who makes them, and several other areas have benefited from systematic bioethical analysis at the federal level (U.S. Congress, 1993). This has typically involved surveying the relevant science, gathering relevant facts, and funneling these inputs into a deliberative process intended to produce a group consensus statement about what principles should guide action. The entire process entails managing all three varieties of uncertainty—scientific and technical, factual, and moral—but analyzing them separately to the degree that is possible.

INFORMED CONSENT IN PSYCHIATRIC GENETICS

The underlying premise of much modern psychiatric research is that mental illness affects the brain. Mental illnesses are similar to other medical conditions in that they can be traced to a causal network of factors that cause deviation from "normal" function. Both biological and social factors are often involved, and indeed interact in complex ways. One of the central tasks of psychiatric research is to tease apart the various factors associated with different psychiatric conditions. One of the central tenets of psychiatric genetics is that genes influence brain function to a measurable degree, and that genetic differences are an important part of the causal network that produces psychiatric disability. As other chapters in this volume amply attest, hunting for genetic factors does not imply that other factors are unimportant; identifying genetic factors will often point to nongenetic factors that interact with genes to cause disability.

Those studying psychiatric conditions must contend not only with the usual problems encountered in other parts of medicine, but also additional problems distinctive to mental disorders. Some of these make the research more technically difficult; others complicate the moral equation. Mental disorders by definition affect the capacities that underlie informed consent to participation in research. Uncertainty about the biological validity of the diagnostic classifications used in psychiatry, fluctuations over time in expression of symptoms, and interdependence of genetic factors with environmental triggers (as, for example, among the addictions, where an environmental factor is part of a disorder's definition) all affect not only the intellectual substance of psychiatric genetics but also the ethical constraints necessary when studying it. Technical and ethical questions cannot be cleanly dissected apart in many cases, but for purposes of first analysis, they can be considered separately.

The moral concern most central to genetic studies in psychiatry is respect for the person who volunteers to participate in research, specifically as that respect is expressed through the process of informed consent. The guidebook used by Institutional Review Boards contains a chapter devoted to "special classes of subjects," which includes a section on "cognitively impaired" persons (Office of Protection from Research Risks, 1993). Most of the points apply not only to cognitive impairment but also equally to disorders of mood, emotion, and perception. In the framework laid out by Faden and Beauchamp, informed consent includes competence to make

choices, sufficient information and understanding of the meaning of participation (risks, benefits, and study rationale, among other things), and voluntariness of choice (Faden & Beauchamp, 1986). Competence is treated as
a threshold, although the legal and moral thresholds may be different. In
contrast, the other two factors—the degree of understanding and freedom
from coercion—lie on continua. Many but not all psychiatric disorders
entail cognitive disabilities that can make understanding difficult, and most
disorders include emotional and affective disabilities that make interpreting
what is understood even more difficult than the study of diabetes or cancer
or heart disease. Serious psychiatric conditions make those who have them
more dependent on family, friends, and social systems, and thus more prone
to coercion. The issue of competence is confused by different meanings
and the potential for distance between legal notions of guardianship and
the authority for others to make decisions on behalf of a person, on the
one hand, and moral precepts of autonomy, on the other. Most of those
suffering from psychiatric conditions are competent to make most decisions,
including decisions about participating in research; but some clearly are
not, and this can produce hard cases and raises many questions about
whether and how to proceed. This is less prominent in psychiatric genetics,
where the purpose of a study is most often to understand the underlying
biology, than in studies of experimental therapy, where research may offer
the possibility of direct benefit to the individual.

Psychiatric disabilities that complicate the informed consent process
have long been recognized as distinctively difficult, along with impairments
associated with mental retardation, dementia, and other conditions with
cognitive and behavioral consequences. A concern that investigators might
exploit those with psychiatric conditions lay behind a 1978 study by the
National Commission for the Protection of Human Subjects of Biomedical
and Behavioral Research. Congress specifically identified three "vulnerable" populations in the National Research Act of 1974 (Public Law 93-
348), which created the National Commission. Each of these special groups
became the subject of a report by the National Commission.

The National Commission recommended a three-tiered system with
special protections for those institutionalized as mentally impaired. The
awkward terminology "those institutionalized as mentally infirm" came
directly from the congressional mandate, combined with the commission's
desire to include not only those who were impaired, but also those deemed
to be so impaired (whether or not there were objective grounds for being
so treated).

The National Commission stipulated several general criteria for studies
that would fall within moral boundaries. It made provisos for solid scientific
background (usually including prior animal studies or other indication of

safety and probable efficacy) and the qualifications of the investigators. The Commission recommended that studies go forward only if there were no way other than involving those institutionalized as mentally infirm. General guidelines for confidentiality came with an exhortation to be vigilant because of the serious problem of stigma attached to many psychiatric conditions, mental retardation, and other conditions affecting brain function. Research should in no circumstances impede health care. For studies that presented "minimal risk," studies could go forward with (1) informed consent of the subject, if possible; (2) if not competent to consent, then a proviso that the research be relevant to the patient's condition and assent obtained; or (3) if no assent were possible or the subject objected, then the research must hold the prospect of direct benefit to that subject (or presence of a monitoring procedure for his or her well-being) and obtain explicit court authorization to proceed. The notion of "assent" for those deemed not legally competent was a novel contribution, creating a duty to communicate even where the law would not otherwise require it.

Research presenting more than minimal risk would require the prospect of direct benefit to the subject (or a monitoring procedure for his or her well-being), the absence of a better alternative treatment, and either consent by the subject or a formal authorization by a court-appointed guardian. Research entailing a "minor increase over minimal risk" was permissible if it were of "vital importance for the understanding or amelioration of the type of disorder or condition of the subjects" or "reasonably expected to benefit" them in the future. This "minor increase over minimal risk" also required an IRB-appointed monitor to follow the study, a procedure that was optional for the lower risk categories. Increasing risk brought increased monitoring. Any override of a patient's objection to participation triggered a requirement for explicit court authorization.

Commissioner Patricia King objected to the recommendation for court involvement to override a subject's objections. She believed that the court was not necessarily best positioned to verify the validity of an objection to research that held the prospect of direct benefit to the patient. She urged that the Commission either not permit an override of objections at all, or that it recommend a different process that might involve the courts but would not necessarily do so. She argued that the process for overriding objections to research that might benefit the particular patient, and available only in the context of such research, should be delegated to the IRB, an IRB-appointed monitor, or both. The IRB or monitor might invoke the courts, but court involvement should not be a requirement.

As it turns out, details of the recommendations were overshadowed by what happened after the National Commission's report was issued. In the other reports on vulnerable populations, such as prisoners and children, recommendations of the National Commission were translated into language for regulations governing federal oversight of experiments involving human subjects (Code of Federal Regulations, 1989). The National Commission's report, including its recommendations for "research involving those institutionalized as mentally infirm," were published in the March 17, 1978, *Federal Register* (U.S. Department of Health, 1978b). Proposed regulations for those deemed "mentally disabled" (the minor change in terminology reflecting comments of the National Commission report) were published on November 17, 1978 (U.S. Department of Health, 1978b), similar to the process for other National Commission reports on vulnerable populations. Unlike the other proposed regulations, however, these were never formally adopted.

The proposed regulations noted uncertainty about how to deal with the question of participation by those not deemed legally competent to give consent (suggesting an appointed monitor might be made mandatory) and what process to use when overriding a subject's objection to participation despite the prospect of direct benefit available only in the context of the research. It held out four options: (1) barring such participation, (2) permitting such research subject to court authorization and consent by the subject's legal representative, (3) in addition to point 2 above, approval by the Secretary of the Department of Health, Education, and Welfare, or (4) in addition to point 2, appointing an "advocate" for the research subject to serve as neutral arbiter.

It became impossible to accommodate both those concerned about violating the civil rights of the mentally disabled and those concerned with unduly burdensome constraints on research (Charles McCarthy, Kennedy Institute of Ethics, Georgetown University, personal communication, October 10, 1994). In the end, the proposed regulations became informal guidelines, and authority over the issues was de facto delegated to IRBs with oversight from the federal Office of Protection from Research Risks. In effect, this left IRBs to make their own determinations under the more general provisions of human subjects protections. Psychiatric conditions and mental retardation were used as case examples and in the IRB Guidebook and other materials that were used to help clarify the meaning of the regulations for IRBs, but the proposed Subpart E of the Code of Federal Regulations was never formally promulgated, nor was it ever withdrawn.

Issues regarding participation in psychiatric research have come up from time to time over the past two decades. In recent years, concern appears to have intensified. An entire issue of *The Journal,* published by the California Alliance for the Mentally Ill, was devoted to this topic, and the passions that fuel the many sides of this debate are abundantly evident (Weisburd, 1994). Most of the controversies about informed consent and psychiatric research surround clinical trials of experimental drugs, but many of the same general problems can arise in psychiatric genetic research. The stakes are high.

All agree that the toll of psychiatric disorders is high. Understanding these disorders is thus critically important, but the severity and nature of the impairments also make such research unusually difficult to conduct. One source of uncertainty is lingering moral disagreement. Research involving human subjects must be conducted in compliance with federal guidelines. Yet federal regulations governing those with psychiatric disabilities have never been made clear, despite considerable effort, because of political and intellectual disagreements. Those disagreements persist. The time for renewed analysis of ethical issues in psychiatric research appears to be at hand. The remainder of this chapter suggests some ways that that analysis might proceed, and how the federal government might begin to resolve the thorny problems.

Two observations about the National Commission report of 1978 are in order, however, before moving on to the special problems of genetics. First, the National Commission report arose from concerns about abuses in institutions—mainly psychiatric hospitals and homes for the mentally retarded. The process of "deinstitutionalization" was already well under way when the National Commission issued its report. Deinstitutionalization had already begun to reduce the population in state psychiatric hospitals and to increase the population in nursing homes, but it had not yet reached a steady state. Clinical trials and other studies were already beginning to move into general hospitals, outpatient clinics, and settings other than mental institutions. The Commission noted this trend, and extended its recommendations to include those who resided outside institutions but were retained on their census. This still excluded a sizable fraction of those with psychiatric conditions, however, who might be involved in research.

In addition to this practical limitation, there is also a conceptual problem. The presumption that institutions are inherently more coercive is not always true. Opportunities for coercion exist wherever there is dependency, and it is not safe to assume that homes or other "noninstitutional" settings are in all cases noncoercive or even less coercive than traditional mental facilities (which differ considerably among themselves). The problem of informed consent in an institutional setting is real, but it does not disappear by walking out the door. A contemporary analysis would necessarily go beyond state mental hospitals and nursing homes to include the special issues that arise in research conducted in home care, foster care, clinics, outpatient services, and other settings.

Several factors have also changed dramatically since the National Commission report. First, the knowledge base and scale of biomedical research have both expanded enormously. Treatments are more effective and more widely available than they were in the 1970s. The busiest two decades in the history of biomedical research lie between us today and the deliberations of the National Commission. Many of the facts uncovered during that period are relevant to the ethical analysis. But perhaps the most important change is dissolution of a consensus about how to regard participation of subjects in research.

The change was signaled most prominently in the context of AIDS treatments. Most of the debate about human subjects in research during the 1960s and 1970s centered on keeping in check the propensity of a few investigators to exploit vulnerable human research subjects. When considering who should be involved first in experiments, for example, Hans Jonas argued that those with good education and high social and economic status should be the first to take risks by participating in research, because they were most likely to appreciate the risks and underlying rationale (Jonas, 1969). This was not mere elitism, but an attempt to codify truly informed consent and to shield more "vulnerable" groups who might not have the same range of free choices as those with more education and resources.

Along the same lines, ethicist Paul Ramsey wrote one of the seminal works of bioethics, *The Patient as Person* (Ramsey, 1970). Ramsey believed that a surrogate should not be able to consent in research that entailed risk for someone else. Taken to its logical conclusion, Ramsey's dictum would preclude surrogate consent for clinical trials. Such studies always entail the risk of untoward side effects, although sufficient direct evidence of likely benefit might overcome this concern. In many early trials, however, the evidence for direct benefit is often highly speculative. Concern about surrogate consent is central for conditions such as Alzheimer's disease, for example, and the cautious voice of Paul Ramsey can be heard in the background even when he is not directly cited (Melnick & Dubler, 1985; Dickens, 1990; Glass & Somerville, 1990; Karlinsky & Lennox, 1990; Kapp, 1994; Marson, Schmitt, Ingram, & Harrell, 1994).

Contrast Ramsey's caution and Jonas's preference for the early involvement of the monied and educated to prevent exploitation with the debate that surrounded early trials of drugs to treat AIDS (Levi, 1991). Here, the opportunity to participate in research was regarded as a benefit to be fought for. The traditional focus of bioethics was turned on its head, replacing fear of exploitation with suspicion that the wealthy and educated will have undue privileges, whereas participation in clinical trials, especially publicly funded ones, should be an entitlement. The bone of contention was not who should be excluded to prevent exploitation, but instead who should be included to ensure fair access. The contemporary scene has both conceptions of research participation contending with one another simultaneously, neither obviously able to trump the other consistently. Revisiting the issues surrounding psychiatric research will not jettison concerns for civil liberties and protection of research subjects' rights such as those expressed by the National Commission in 1978, but additional rights will surely be debated, and the direction policy should take is not transparently clear.

HOW THE HUMAN GENOME PROJECT HAS DEALT WITH ETHICAL CONCERNS

In addition to the problems that beset any research involving those with impaired mental capacities, another set of ethical issues arise in connection with genetic research. The federal government is addressing these ethical issues largely through a research program made part of the Human Genome Project.

The Human Genome Project, which officially began in 1990, is the result of the growing importance of genetics in biomedical research. The Project, actually a collection of loosely linked scientific initiatives in many different countries and international organizations, grew out of technological progress in methods directly to study DNA. The Human Genome Project is primarily an effort to construct research tools—to build the informational and technological infrastructure for human genetic studies. The output of the Human Genome Project—maps, methods, databases, and instruments—is intended to be an input for studies of conditions that run in families. In psychiatric genetics, this means that the technical aspects of studies will be improved, so that the molecular biology and its analysis will be faster and more precise.

In the vigorous debate that accompanied the genesis of the Human Genome Project, examination of the ethical, legal, and social implications of the new knowledge emerged as an additional goal. At a press conference in September to announce his appointment as head of the new NIH Office of Human Genome Research, James Watson declared his intention to devote a fraction of the genome research budget to study the ethical implications of genome science and its applications (Watson, 1988). The importance of looking at the broader social and legal implications of genome research had been identified in the two major policy reports released earlier that year (National Research Council, 1988; U.S. Congress, 1988). Neither of these reports was specific about how to accomplish this, however, and Watson decided to take the lead in the NIH genome project rather than merely assume it would be carried on somewhere else.

NIH began its Ethical, Legal, and Social Implications (ELSI) program be delegating its steerage to a working group chaired by Nancy S. Wexler. Wexler was a psychologist long associated with the genetic approach to Huntington's disease, and a major figure in a private charity founded by her father, the Hereditary Disease Foundation. The working group met for the first time in September, 1989, and laid out a set of themes for research to be supported by the program, using NIH's usual mechanisms of grants and contracts. Following strong pressure from Senator Albert Gore, Jr., at a November, 1989, hearing (U.S. Senate, 1989), the Department of Energy followed suit. The ELSI fraction of the NIH genome budget increased from 3% to 5% between 1990 and 1992, at which point the 5% figure became mandated by the NIH authorization statute. The fraction at DOE remained at 3%. This approach to scientific responsibility—directly attaching a research program on social implications to a scientific and technical initiative—was unprecedented.

The roots of the ELSI program lay not in the project itself, but in the social history of human genetics more broadly, most notably its prominence in the social policy movements that were known as eugenics during the first several decades of this century and the recombinant DNA controversy of the 1970s. Even as the idea of a genome project was being hatched, a renascent field of scholarship on the eugenics movement was gathering steam. Daniel Kevles's pioneering book on the American and British eugenics movements (Kevles, 1985) was soon followed by many others. Robert Jay Lifton looked at the role of the Nazi doctors, and Robert Proctor analyzed the role of German scientists and physicians on the racial hygiene movement that culminated in the Holocaust (Lifton, 1986; Proctor, 1988). Proctor devoted a section of his book to the transition from eugenics, associated with the first deliberate killings of psychiatric patients, and how it only later became linked to racial hygiene, when the same facilities designed to exterminate those whose lives were "not worth living" were available for use on Jews, Gypsies, and others. This is a particularly grotesque illustration of the dangers of a too facile imputation of psychiatric illness to genetic factors. The elimination of psychiatric patients was not solely or even mainly premised on genetics. Another main line of argument was to reduce the fiscal drag of the psychiatrically impaired on the rest of society. Genetic arguments were nonetheless a part of the complex of factors that culminated in heinous excesses. Mark Adams studied the eugenics movements in many different nations, and noted their heterogeneity and uniqueness, but also documented the worldwide currency of genetic ideas about socially esteemed or reviled human characteristics (Adams, 1990).

A postwar generation of American geneticists was trained with little explicit attention to the history of eugenics, only dimly aware of the degree to which eugenics was linked to the early history of their field. The scholars of eugenics changed this dramatically, so that most of those being trained in medical genetics and genetic counseling now learn about eugenics.

The discovery of recombinant DNA in the mid-1970s also exposed many public fears about too rapid application of the "new biology" (Krimsky, 1982). When scientists imposed a moratorium on their own work, it demonstrated a willingness to behave responsibly, but the intense debate among scientists, politicians, social critics, and activists of various stripes left a permanent residue of discomfiture with the power of molecular genetics. In the early to mid-1980s, the prospect of human gene therapy—the deliberate treatment of diseases by introducing DNA into patients—rekindled this debate.

The federal government had sponsored bioethics through grants under the Ethics and Values in Science program at the National Science Foundation (NSF) and grants from the National Endowment for the Humanities (NEH). The NSF program was intended to cover ethical issues arising in science and technology, a very broad mandate, and a principal criterion of the NEH program was to advance work in the humanities. The purpose of the genome ELSI program was more focused, with an explicit linkage to social policy. The ELSI program was intended primarily to foster benefits and thwart misuses of human genetic research, not to study values in science nor to advance the humanities and social science.

The ELSI program had two major components: a research program and the working group which helped steer the research program but also had duties to translate the research into options for policymakers. In the research program, most support went to university-based projects funded through competitively reviewed grants. Some of the Department of Energy funds went to support work at the national laboratories, most notably a privacy-centered project at Los Alamos National Laboratory. DOE focused its effort on privacy, employment-related concerns, and education. The larger NIH program included these, but devoted even more resources to how clinically relevant genetic research was conducted and how genetic tests were introduced into clinical practice. There were several other program elements, ranging from the practicalities of DNA forensics to very basic philosophical inquiry about the meaning of genetic information and issues of justice concerning its use.

Most elements of the ELSI program are relevant to psychiatric genetics, but two areas are particularly instructive. The first concerns the conduct of family studies, especially relevant to genetic linkage studies, one main theme in psychiatric genetics. The second area, a cluster of studies focused on the events that take place after a gene is discovered, illustrates how empirical studies might improve policy decisions.

The tradition of family studies in genetics dated back roughly a half century. The field was a relatively small part of biomedical research for several decades. The genetic approach to diseases of unknown cause was given a big boost when David Botstein and his colleagues laid out how a global genetic linkage map might be made for the human chromosomes, and gave examples of the immense power of such a map (Botstein, White, Skolnick, & Davis, 1980). This approach had its first major success in 1983, by identifying the chromosome region containing the gene that causes Huntington's disease (Gusella *et al.,* 1983). Over the next half decade, this strategy of establishing genetic linkage was successful for dozens of other diseases, and became widely accepted as a promising approach to disorders that were known to run in families but whose biology was otherwise mysterious.

The availability of tools to expedite genetic linkage of many diseases meant more families were being studied. Studies in families raised ethical issues at each stage of the research. Just contacting an individual in a family affected by a disorder could be tricky. Information within families is not always freely shared, and this is especially true when conditions are associated with shame and stigma. The fact that a grandmother or grandfather or cousin or aunt or uncle was affected with breast cancer or Alzheimer's disease or schizophrenia might be hidden. The fact that genetic research was being undertaken might be taken as proof that investigators thought the disease in question was inherited in one's own family. A Minnesota study of breast cancer undertaken in the 1950s was an early indication that some cases might be influenced by genetic factors. When investigators decided to follow up on this study by contacting the relatives of affected women, to track the inheritance in families (and lack of inheritance in others), it turned out that over 26% of the women had no knowledge of the family history of breast cancer. Although the vast majority of first-degree relatives (siblings and children) knew, 27% of second degree and more than half of third-degree relatives did not know (T. A. Sellers, personal communication).

The act of initial contact had several major potential impacts. First, it disclosed a risk that was hitherto unknown, and a particularly fearsome prospect of breast cancer in this case. The information was potentially quite disruptive, but might be delivered before investigators had any agreement to participate in a study. In addition, this information could put women in awkward situations. When seeking private insurance and in some other contexts, individuals are often asked questions about family history. Before contact from the investigators, women could truthfully state they had no knowledge of a family history of cancer. After contact, they might be in the position of either having to lie about their family history or saying "yes" to a family history of cancer. This might put their access to private insurance at risk. Mere contact for participation in a study, therefore, might cause both psychological harm and put individuals at risk of discrimination when seeking private insurance and employment.

While many or even most women might welcome the new information because they simply wanted to know information pertinent to their health or because it enabled closer medical monitoring and earlier intervention in the event of actually developing cancer, they could also be put at psychological and social risk. The fact that investigators were studying breast cancer in families could pit medical benefit against social harm, forcing judgments that individuals should be able to make themselves as a conscious choice to participate or not in research. It was possible to design a study to avoid inadvertent disclosure of potentially damaging information by broadening the sample to include nonfamilial cases and being careful in what was disclosed at time of initial contact. But such careful studies required ample forethought. Such forethought was by no means routine, and an initial study of IRBs, even those at centers of genetics, were largely oblivious to the issues involved (Peter Weir, presentation to ELSI Working Group, Bethesda, December 5, 1994).

Once a study were under way, family studies introduced complexities not confronted to the same degree when doing studies of unrelated individuals. Information about one person gave information about others in the same family. Moreover, getting informative data on one person might require getting others in the same family to participate. Establishing genetic linkage of a disease, for example, depended on being able to trace the inheritance of chromosome markers through families. Sometimes the genetic constitution of a "skipped" individual could be inferred, at other times it could not. When it could not, giving useful information to those related to a critical person in the pedigree would depend on his or her agreement to participate in the study. This could be especially important in psychiatric genetic studies, because the emotional toll of the disorders is quite high, and the likelihood of family conflict may also be higher.

It was also not clear what it meant to participate or withdraw from a family genetic study. Did every person in a family have to consent? What would it mean for a person to object to a study? If a critical person in a pedigree objected, would that imply that his or her marker profile should not be reconstructed, regardless of the impact on others in the family? What if someone agreed to participate but then pulled out? Should all records be pulled, or should the genetic data already in place be left for the benefit of others in the family, but no new information added? What about the clinical information that made the genetic data useful? What would happen when a grant ran out but the data were still of great value to the family? Did the family or the investigator own and control the data?

Many of these questions emanated from the distinctively collective nature of genetic data. Most bioethical analysis had proceeded under the assumption of a dyadic relationship between individuals and investigators. In family studies, the investigator was simultaneously attached to multiple family members whose information could affect others in the same family.

These issues had always attended family studies, but they began to receive more attention under the ELSI program. An early grant to the American Association for the Advancement of Science focused attention on the issues. At a March, 1992, workshop in Charleston, South Carolina, a group of genetic researchers, policy analysts, bioethicists, and others assembled to discuss the novel issues arising in family studies (Frankel & Teich, 1993). Discussion at the workshop was based in large part on several case studies presented by those directly engaged in pedigree studies of different kinds of disorders. One of the most complex case studies was contributed by Sylvia Simpson of Johns Hopkins University, who discussed manic-depressive disorder (Simpson, 1993). This workshop was followed up by a subsequent NIH-sponsored meeting that raised serious concerns about privacy and confidentiality issues, and became the basis for a new section on genetic studies in the guidebook prepared for IRBs (Office of Protection from Research Risks, 1993). The ELSI program thus focused attention on an aspect of research ethics that lay at the heart of genetic research but had been relatively neglected.

NIH and DOE both funded an Institute of Medicine study, *Assessing Genetic Risks,* among their first ELSI program contracts. The report came out early in 1994, and became the largest and most comprehensive study of the issues surrounding the use of genetic tests in an era when genetics was becoming more important in many aspects of medical care. The committee that prepared the report urged "caution in the use and interpretation of presymptomatic or predictive tests" in particular, and noted "if predictive tests for mental disorders become a reality, results must be handled with stringent attention to confidentiality to protect an already vulnerable population" (Andrews, Fullarton, Holtzman, & Motulsky, 1994). One paragraph of that report focused on psychiatric disorders, and makes points directly relevant not only to clinical use of tests, but also to studies in the research phase:

> It is likely that multiple genes, often interacting with yet poorly understood
> environmental factors, will be operative in many psychiatric disorders. As with
> other complex conditions, predictive testing in psychiatric diseases is unlikely

to be as accurate as prediction in monogenic diseases (those caused by a single gene of major effect). Prediction will always be more probabilistic, and there will be uncertainty regarding whether the disorder will ever manifest and, if so, at what age. The implications of predictive testing for mental disorders raise even more problems than those for other complex medical diseases, because of the heightened potential for stigmatization and discrimination. [Andrews *et al.*, 1994]

The ELSI program began by funding conferences, workshops, and a few policy studies. Its most distinctive contribution to policy analysis, however, came from turning attention to empirical studies of practices in research and medical care. This opened a particularly promising avenue for fruitful inquiry in bioethics, moving it from a purely theoretical and deliberative field to one also grounded in creating new information relevant to policy decisions. Empirical ELSI studies came about in large part as a response to the advance of genetics, in particular the discovery of disease-related genes.

The first wave of enthusiasm for the Human Genome Project was fueled by the spate of successes in finding genetic linkage to several disorders in the period 1985–1988. These early successes in genetic linkage owed relatively little to the Human Genome Project, except significant overlap in intellectual ancestry. The second wave came when genetic linkage, yielding the approximate location of a gene but not the gene itself, gave way to successful gene hunts that turned up the genes themselves. The work to find a gene following linkage could be considerable. In the case of Huntington's disease, for example, it took a full decade of work by a large collaborative group to move from linkage in 1983 to discovery of a mutation in 1993 (Huntington's Disease Collaborative Research Group, MacDonald *et al.*, 1993).

The genetic strategy of disease association, hunting for a specific gene and then working toward function and biochemistry rather than the reverse, had its first success with chronic granulomatous disease (Royer *et al.*, 1987) and Duchenne muscular dystrophy (Koenig *et al.*, 1987). But these conditions had long been known to reside on the X chromosome. Cystic fibrosis (CF) was a relatively common genetic disorder, affecting roughly one in 3500 children or over 1000 births per year in the United States. The location of its gene was completely unknown, and the underlying biology was quite mysterious, with many theories but none fully elaborated in molecular detail. When CF was linked to a small region on chromosome 7 in 1985 (Tsui *et al.*, 1985; Wainwright *et al.*, 1985; White *et al.*, 1985), it was a major breakthrough, and this led 4 years later to the gene itself (Kerem *et al.*, 1989; Riordan *et al.*, 1989; Rommens *et al.*, 1989). The nature of the gene and its resultant protein gave strong clues about its function as a molecular channel for chloride ions to flow through cell membranes, already suspected on biochemical grounds but now confirmed with wondrous molecular precision with gene and protein in hand. The defect could be corrected in cells by replacing a defective gene with a normal copy, showing the power of having genetic clues to guide further biological studies, and even suggesting the eventual possibility of gene therapy (Rich *et al.*, 1990).

Finding a gene was a great scientific advance. It also marked a transition from one phase of application to another. In disorders for which only linkage in families had been available for diagnosis, for example, having a gene enabled them now to specify a specific mutation and analyze DNA directly. In cases where the mutation was known and the relation between gene and disease straightforward, this led directly to a diagnostic test. Most disorders, including Huntington's disease and CF, proved to be more complex than imagined at first. The degree of variation at the genetic level, with many different mutations in the same gene, far exceeded expectations. While this complicated diagnostic testing, DNA-based diagnosis was nonetheless powerfully aided by having a known gene to analyze.

When the CF gene was discovered in 1989, the first reaction was euphoria. It was a resounding success, having in half a decade transited the full course from a fairly common disease whose molecular cause was largely unknown through genetic linkage and then finding a gene to identification of a molecular function—an astonishing success in many regards. Even as the gene was discovered, speculation turned to what it would mean for diagnosis and ultimately treatment. After a few months, speculation gave way to some concern about what to do about DNA-based diagnosis. Concern grew from two independent sources, technical and ethical. On the technical side, the number of different ways to mutate the same gene began to seem unending. The number of new mutations did not stop at 100 or 200 or even 300; it kept on going up. There were a few mutations that accounted for the majority of cases in most populations (the Northern European populations were the simplest to analyze, with the least variety of different ones).

It became obvious in the early months that in most populations, a DNA test for CF would need to measure several mutations, and in the rare family it would be difficult and expensive indeed until the technologies for simultaneously testing hundreds of mutations at once were possible. At the time, such technologies were only a speculative prospect. Finding the gene was a major boon within families known to be at risk, because the birth of an affected child signaled the presence of mutations in both mother and father, and the child's CF gene could be analyzed directly to see which mutations were present in that particular family (to see if they were both among the half dozen fairly common ones, and hence easily tested, or rarer mutations requiring more work to analyze). When screening a population, however, a much more sensitive and specific test was needed or it risked missing many cases, giving false reassurance to a few families at risk and not giving definitive answers to many families identified as possibly at risk (when one parent had a known mutation but the other parent tested normal). One major concern was the potential demand for populationwide screening in the face of the test's insensitivity. Another was that potential profit would entice testing laboratories to market the tests prematurely. The first warning came in November 1989, when the American Society of Human Genetics issued a statement (Caskey, Ka-back, & Beaudet, 1990).

Ethical concerns grew from the population frequency of CF, the most common single-gene disorder of children with recessive inheritance (mean-ing a child got the disease only when he or she inherited a CF mutant gene on chromosome 7 from *both* the mother and father, not just one or the other). A 1983 report of the President's Commission for the Study of Ethical Problems in Medicine and Biomedical and Behavioral Research, *Screening and Counseling for Genetic Conditions,* had devoted a chapter to the drain that a genetic test for CF might place on the nation's small and fragile network of genetic services (President's Commission, 1983c).

At its second meeting in Williamsburg, Virginia, in February of 1990, the ELSI working group identified "tracking the cystic fibrosis experience" as its number one priority (Fink, 1990). NIH convened a workshop on CF testing the next month, sponsored by the genome center and five other NIH units. Planning for this meeting was already well under way when the ELSI working group met, under the leadership of Nancy Lamontagne of the Cystic Fibrosis Program at the National Institute of Diabetes and Diges-tive and Kidney Diseases (NIDDK). The NIH workshop also cautioned about premature genetic screening and noted that pilot studies of CF testing as a prelude to widespread use were "urgently needed" (NIH Workshop on Population Screening for the Cystic Fibrosis Gene, 1990).

Money did not follow good intentions. The only grant reviewed on CF testing that year was rejected by a peer review group on specious grounds (Cook-Deegan, 1994), and trepidation about getting caught in the divisive abortion debate paralyzed the Cystic Fibrosis Foundation and NIDDK (Roberts, 1990). The ELSI program and the NIH genome center, however, crashed forward. The November meeting of the ELSI working group considered a paper by University of Wisconsin physicians Benjamin Wilfond and Norman Fost that pointed to potential problems in CF testing (Wilfond & Fost, 1990), and urged that the ELSI program support pilot projects even if other institutes at NIH would not. In December, the genome center's outside advisory committee endorsed a resolution to move forward with CF testing (NCHGR Program Advisory Committee on the Human Genome, 1990), despite concerns that it might consume a large share of the ELSI program funds. By the end of January, staff directed by Eric Juengst of the genome center had organized a workshop to help frame a call for grant proposals. The request for applications was issued in April (National Center for Human Genome Research, National Center for Nursing Research *et al.,* 1991), and the awards to seven institutions announced in October (National Center for Human Genome Research, 1990). Funding came from the genome center, the nursing center, and the child health institute at NIH (NIDDK, parent of the CF research program, was notably absent). This expeditious movement was truly awesome compared to the usual progress of new initiatives at NIH.

The investigators funded by these grants met the next month to agree on terms that would enable some comparisons among studies but also allow different studies to focus on different aspects and clinical scenarios for testing (Lawson, 1991). In addition to the suite of studies supported by NIH, the Department of Energy also supported a project that directly compared families tested for sickle-cell disease to those tested for CF, trying to use both quantitative and qualitative sociological methods to study differences among African-Americans and Caucasians, and to tease them apart from differences associated with income and social standing, under the direction of Troy Duster and Diane Beeson, based at the University of California, Berkeley.

These empirical studies turned up several surprising facts. The demand was not as overwhelming as many had feared. It was highly dependent on when and how a test was offered (Andrews, 1993). The sociological study made it clear that women were the main arbiters of genetic information in families of all stripes. There was far greater suspicion of the motives of those doing the testing, less optimism about benefits from testing, and lower hopes of finding a technical fix for the disease among families seeking sickle cell testing; a second phase of research attempted to tease apart ethnic from social and economic factors (Beeson, 1993). Preliminary data from the studies indicated how education affected demand for the interpretation of tests, identified some problems among different groups offering the tests, noted some effects of the complexity of the informed consent process in the families seeking testing, and demonstrated that use was quite sensitive to price. An interim report concluded that programs started without the data coming from the pilot studies might well "have been inappropriately designed" (Andrews, 1993). Just as important, the grants program fostered an evidentiary and rational approach to a new and highly complex technology that was producing highly nuanced and immensely personal information for families facing important decisions, in stark contrast to the willy-nilly introduction of many other medical technologies (Wilfond & Nolan, 1993).

Even as the CF studies were yielding useful data, the research community was turning up genes associated with many different kinds of cancer. Some genes were associated with multiple forms of cancer. In other cases, multiple genes were associated with a single form of cancer. A flood of studies commenced in the mid-1980s, with discovery of the gene causing a rare eye cancer, retinoblastoma, that in some cases was inherited as a genetic trait (Cavenee *et al.*, 1985; Friend *et al.*, 1986; Lee *et al.*, 1987). The deluge of cancer gene discoveries intensified. A gene that coded for protein p53 was found to explain the very high risk in "cancer families." They were prone to cancer in many organs starting in childhood, and having the gene in hand raised serious questions about whom to test and when (Li, 1992). The discovery of two genes for colon cancer and one of two known for breast cancer brought the immediacy of genetics and cancer to much more common disorders.

The success in pilot studies of CF genetic tests made a similar effort in cancer gene testing appealing. A consortium of projects was again pulled together with multiple NIH institutes, this time focused on testing for the most common cancers whose genes had been identified: breast, ovarian, and colon cancers. The NIH genome center was joined by the National Cancer Institute, the National Institute of Mental Health, and the National Institute on Nursing Research in a request for applications announced in February, 1994 (National Center for Human Genome Research, 1994), with $2.5 million in awards made to 11 projects that fall (Anonymous, 1994).

The pilot testing programs were by far the largest cluster of grants in the ELSI portfolio, accounting for a large majority of the NIH's portfolio of ELSI grants in 1992 through 1994. There were other studies under way. In early years, the ELSI program had funded many conferences that were general, and became important in outreach and in helping set the policy agenda. After 2 years, however, conference grants became quite difficult to secure, replaced by more focused research efforts from many different disciplines. As the CF and then cancer testing pilot projects got under way, these research grants got squeezed in the funding competition, reaching a nadir in 1994, when only 1 of 39 grant applications coming through the general program announcement was funded (as opposed to responding to the request for cancer testing pilot projects or "education" grants, which were reviewed separately) (Thomson & Drell, 1995). After 5 years, the ELSI grants program had become more competitive and more tightly funded than the general grants program in the genome center, and among the most competitive grant programs at NIH and DOE. At NIH's genome center, 39% of the grant applications were for the ELSI program, yet it accounted for only 5% of the funding. This was apt to prove sufficiently discouraging to most investigators to cause a backlash, with a large store of ill feelings, because even the luminaries of the various fields were unlikely to be funded. The ELSI program had proved that if funding were available, the grant applications would come. But they grew much faster than the funds.

The ELSI program had some secondary effects that were predictable, but unavoidable and not really its fault. The main untoward impact within bioethics was to strongly skew the research agenda of biomedical ethics in the direction of genetics. Genetics did not come to completely dominate bioethics because of even larger body of work centered on health care decisions and practices in clinics and hospitals (the branch of medical ethics). In ethical analysis related to research, however, genetics did come to dominate the scene. The problem here was not that the ELSI program existed, but that similar programs in other fields did not.

The ELSI program changed the face of bioethics, mainly for the better. It provided much more funding for research in a focused area than had ever been available anywhere before. It provided a formal peer review system with sufficient volume to generate some consistency. And it merged bioethics with disciplines not only engaged in deliberation and fact-filtering, such as history and philosophy, but also of data creation and direct empirical inquiry. This was enormously powerful and useful, and a major innovation. But how would all this research and other work translate into policy?

One salient weakness in the ELSI program was related to its own configuration—the difficulty in turning facts and studies into tools useful for making policy decisions (Roberts, 1993). The ELSI program was highly successful in funding solid work; it was less clear how well its second mission, translating that work into policy, was being carried out. Certainly the data generated from the program were of great relevance to those making policy decisions. Over time, this might even find its way into the policy process at all levels. Within the genetics community, publication in a technical journal or even mention at a meeting might be sufficient to help change policies at the institutions near the cutting edge. In some cases, there were connections to state government, either through legislators or state administrations, and new policies could be fostered locally. But the ELSI program was a national program, and the main standard for success would be measured at the federal level, by impact on new laws, regulations, and on national professional and scientific groups. To expedite progress at the federal level, however, it appeared the ELSI program would need a boost.

FEDERAL BIOETHICS COMMISSIONS

Bioethics had provided several models for policy impact at the federal level, and several examples of failure. The two most notable successes were federal bioethics commissions: the National Commission for the Protection of Human Subjects of Biomedical and Behavioral Research (National Commission), which operated from late 1974 through 1978, and the President's Commission for the Study of Ethical Problems in Medicine and Biomedical and Behavioral Research (the President's Commission), which operated between 1980 and 1983. The National Commission, whose report on those institutionalized as mentally infirm was noted above, produced that report and seven others (National Commission, 1975, 1976, 1977a–c, 1978a–e). Among these was a short paper, *The Belmont Report,* that laid out the principles that guided the National Commission's deliberations, arguably the most influential document in all of contemporary bioethics (National Commission, 1978a). The National Commission—which was widely expected to fail because it was forced to handle explosive issues such as research on prisoners, psychosurgery, and especially fetal research—succeeded in producing reports that were both scholarly and laid out explicit arguments, but also extremely useful. Most of the reports were translated directly into federal regulations governing research that involved people. The move to draw regulations predated the National Commission, but the Commission gave the regulations explicit public justification and the clout that comes from a conspicuous national forum (Faden & Beauchamp, 1986; U.S. Congress, 1993).

The President's Commission was elevated out of the Department of Health Education and Welfare (now known as the Department of Health and Human Services) and made a presidential commission with a somewhat broader mandate. It included research involving people, but also included topics in mainstream health care. The President's Commission also had the power to initiate studies, an important feature distinguishing it from its predecessor. The President's Commission issued 11 reports before its sunset clause took effect (following a 3-month extension) (President's Commission, 1981a,b, 1982a–d, 1983a–e). None of these reports dealt directly with topics in psychiatric genetics, except tangential references in reports on gene therapy (President's Commission, 1982c) and the report on genetic screening and counseling noted in the discussion about CF above (President's Commission, 1983c). The President's Commission cut an even higher profile than the National Commission, and again demonstrated the power of a national forum and staff resources for explicit consideration of hot topics. The reports issued by both the National and President's Commissions remain highly cited in the bioethics literature to this day, and the Commissions influenced statutes and policies at both the state and federal level.

Between the National and President's Commissions, the Ethics Advisory Board existed within the Department of Health, Education and Welfare from 1978 until 1980. It was a combination traffic cop and deliberative body. Its functions included review of specific research proposals that fell outside or at the margin of the human subjects regulations and needed special approval. It was also a national forum for topics related to biomedical research. Its traffic cop role could not be served by the President's Commission, but failure to appreciate the disparate roles led to diverting the Ethics Advisory Board's budget to help launch the President's Commission. The Ethics Advisory Board therefore issued only a few reports and made recommendations to NIH about a research protocol bearing on *in vitro* fertilization, on techniques for visualizing the living fetus, and on a few other matters before passing quietly out of existence (U.S. Congress, 1993).

Success of the President's Commission led to the desire for another federal bioethics commission. The result was the Biomedical Ethics Advisory Committee (BEAC). BEAC was essentially a small congressional agency modeled on the Office of Technology Assessment, with a 12-member bipartisan congressional board—three Democrats and three Republicans from each the House and Senate. The process of appointing the outside advisory committee that would actually oversee operations and do the work proved quite difficult, consuming over 2 years. When one of the members died, the process of replacing him fanned the smoldering coals of abortion politics, and the BEAC flamed out. BEAC met for the first time in September, 1988, and met only once more in February, 1989. BEAC died when its funding was effectively killed for fiscal year 1990 (U.S. Congress, 1993). Other efforts to do bioethics at the national level also foundered during that same period, including a prominent panel looking at the transplantation of fetal cells to study experimental treatments for brain and other disorders (Childress, 1991). That panel's deliberative process was punctuated by several crises, and its majority recommendations were ultimately rejected by the Assistant Secretary of Health, the Secretary of Health, and the Bush Administration. The Clinton administration lifted a ban on such research early in its tenure, however, although a subsequent panel's recommendations were overridden by the President (White House, 1994).

The success of the National and President's Commissions gave hope for the usefulness of a national bioethics forum, but the examples of BEAC and the fetal tissue transplantation panel indicated the difficulties in replicating those successes. The debate about a national bioethics commission was rekindled in December, 1993, when the Office of Technology Assessment hosted a workshop at the request of Senator Mark O. Hatfield. The notion of a bioethics commission attracted bipartisan support in the Senate, sparking serious discussions between Senators Hatfield and Edward M. Kennedy. In the meantime, OTA director Jack Gibbons became the White House science advisor. Vice President Albert Gore, Jr., was also a long-time supporter of bioethics during his previous congressional career in the House and Senate. During 1994, movement toward a bioethics commission took place in both the Senate and Executive Branch. Health care reform ultimately precluded attention to bioethics in Congress, but the White House Office of Science and Technology Policy published the charter for a proposed National Bioethics Advisory Committee (NBAC) on August 12, 1994 (Office of Science and Technology Policy, 1994). On December 2, 1994, President Clinton declared, "In order to ensure that advice on complex bioethical issues that affect our society can continue to be developed, we are planning to move forward with the establishment of a National Bioethics Advisory Commission over the next year" (White House, 1994).

On October 3, 1995, President Clinton issued an Executive Order that created the National Bioethics Advisory Commission (Office of the Press Secretary, 1995). The order accompanied the release of a major report from an external advisory committee that labored for 18 months to study the involvement of human subjects in radiation experiments. The report included a review of human subject protections and pointed to several "outstanding policy issues in need of public resolution," including one of direct relevance here: "Guidelines for research with adults of questionable competence. Of particular concern is more-than-minimal-risk research that offers adults of questionable competence no prospect of offsetting medical benefit" (Advisory Committee on Human Radiation Experiments, 1995, p. 822). The report also cautioned that the distinction between clinical care and research was often blurred, and those participating in research often had unrealistic expectations of direct medical benefit. The President's executive order built on the report's findings, stating "As a first priority, the National Bioethics Advisory Committee shall direct its attention to consideration of protection of the rights and welfare of human research subjects and issues in the management and use of genetic information" (Office of the Press Secretary, 1995).

The proposal to create a new bioethics forum pertains to psychiatric genetics in two respects. First, the charter calls for examination of issues related to human subjects in research. While discussions about a bioethics commission were taking place in 1994, the controversy surrounding antipsychotic drug trials among patients with schizophrenia erupted into the national press. Senator Kennedy and the White House staff were focused on this problem and definitely had it in mind when charting directions for

NBAC (staff of the Senate Labor and Human Resources Committee; staff of the Office of Science and Technology Policy, personal communications with the author, February through November, 1994). The second main mandate in the draft charter focuses on genetic privacy, another primary concern in psychiatric genetics.

CONCLUSIONS

The stage is now set for a more systematic and penetrating approach to bioethics at the federal level, although budget constraints may preclude as much action as would take place otherwise. On the one hand, the ELSI grant program has amply demonstrated the value of a long-term research program that creates new information. When dealing with the controversy over involvement of psychiatric patients in clinical trials, for example, investigators often point to the difficulties of informed consent, and the need to engage in an oral process more than laying a paper trail. When confronted with the same problem, however, a federal office charged with ensuring compliance with human subjects regulations has little to go on but case histories and the documentary record. In the absence of empirical data that bear out investigators' claims, based on direct study of the informed consent process in psychiatric research, the controversy is necessarily a standoff, with strong and appealing arguments on both sides and no data to negotiate the middle ground. The ELSI grants program has demonstrated that empirical studies can address questions of direct concern to the conduct of research and its transition to application. It is well within the mandate of the National Institute of Mental Health, the National Institute on Drug Abuse, the National Institute on Alcohol Abuse and Alcoholism, and other federal research agencies to conduct such studies. Indeed, there have been empirical studies of informed consent in practice and in research, but not at a consistent and sustained level sufficient to advance policy.

Translation into policy in a systematic fashion may be difficult for work sponsored only at the agency level. The ELSI program here indicates great success in influencing the course of research and to some degree the behavior of biomedical research and even medical service constituencies, but success in federal policy change is less apparent. This could be a question of time, of circumstance and opportunity, or of insufficiency of means. It is an open question whether the research program will translate into federal policy on its own, or whether it needs a federal bioethics commission to help it along. The approaches are by no means mutually exclusive, but instead are highly complementary. Indeed, if a national bioethics forum comes into being, the wealth of facts, experts, and prior consideration of the relevant questions will be considerably greater in the areas of human genetics covered by the ELSI program than could be tapped to assist previous bioethics commissions. If the National Bioethics Advisory Committee is created, psychiatric genetics will almost certainly become a subject of its attention, both when addressing the ethics of human subjects in research and when considering the privacy of genetic information.

REFERENCES

Adams, M. B. (Ed.). (1990). *The wellborn science: Eugenics in Germany, France, Brazil, and Russia.* London: Oxford University Press.

Advisory Committee on Human Radiation Experiments. (Release date copy, October 3, 1995). *Final report.* Page numbers may change from final report to be made available as Stock Number 061-000-00-848-9 from the U.S. Government Printing Office, Washington, DC.

Andrews, L. B. (1993, December). *Testing and counseling for cystic fibrosis mutations: An independent contractor report on interim findings.* Working Group on Ethical, Legal, and Social Implications of Genome Research.

Andrews, L. B., Fullarton, J. E., Holtzman, N. A., & Motulsky, A. G. (Ed.). (1994). *Assessing genetic risks: Implications for health and social policy* (pp. 9–10, 106). Washington, DC: National Academy Press.

Anonymous. (1994). NIH grants explore issues related to genetic testing for cancer risk. *Human Genome News, 6*(November), 15.

Beeson, D. (1993, September 9). *Presentation to the working group.* Working Group on Ethical, Legal, and Social Implications of Human Genome Research.

Botstein, D., White, R. L., Skolnick, M., & Davis, R. W. (1980). Construction of a genetic linkage map in man using restriction fragment length polymorphisms. *American Journal of Human Genetics, 32,* 314–331.

Caskey, C. T., Kaback, M. M., & Beaudet, A. L. (1990). The American Society of Human Genetics statement on cystic fibrosis screening. *American Journal of Human Genetics, 46,* 393.

Cavenee, W. K., Hansen, M. F., Nordernskjold, M., *et al.* (1985). Genetic origin of mutations predisposing to retinoblastoma. *Science, 228,* 501–503.

Childress, J. F. (1991). Deliberations of the Human Fetal Tissue Transplantation Research Panel. In K. E. Hanna (Ed.), *Biomedical politics* (pp. 215–248). Washington, DC: National Academy Press.

Code of Federal Regulations, Part 46—Protection of Human Subjects, revised as of March 8, 1983, reprinted July 31, 1989. *Code of Federal Regulations,* Title 45, Section 46; available through the Office of Protection from Research Risks, National Institutes of Health, July 31, 1989.

Cook-Deegan, R. M. (1994). A new social contract. In *The gene wars: Science, politics, and the human genome* (pp. 243–246). New York: Norton.

Dickens, B. M. (1990). Substitute consent to participation of persons with Alzheimer's disease in medical research: Legal issues. In J. M. Berg, H. Karlinsky, & F. Lowy (Eds.), *Alzheimer's disease research: Ethical and legal issues* (pp. 76–90). Toronto: Carswell.

Faden, R. R., & Beauchamp, T. L. (1986). *A history and theory of informed consent.* London: Oxford University Press.

Fink, L. (1990, April 3). Summary: First Workshop of the Joint Working Group on the Ethical, Legal, and Social Issues Related to Mapping and Sequencing the Human Genome. National Center for Human Genome Research.

Frankel, M. S., & Teich, A. H. (Eds.). (1993). *Ethical and legal issues in pedigree research.* Washington, DC: American Association for the Advancement of Science.

Friend, S. H., Bernards, R., Rogelj, S., Weinberg, R. A., Rapaport, J. M., Albert D. M., & Dryja, T. P. (1986). A human DNA segment with properties of the gene that prediposes to retinoblastoma and osteosarcoma. *Nature, 323,* 643–646.

Glass, K. C., & Somerville, M. A. (1990). Informed consent to medical research on persons with Alzheimer's disease: Ethical and legal parameters. In J. M. Berg, H. Karlinsky, & F. Lowy (Eds.), *Alzheimer's disease research: Ethical and legal issues* (pp. 30–59). Toronto: Carswell.

Gusella, J. F., Wexler, N. S., Conneally, P. M., Naylor, S. L., Anderson, M. A., Tanzi, R. E., Watkind, P. C., Ottina, K., Wallace, M. R., Sakaguchi, A. Y., Young, A. M., Shoulson, I., Bonilla, E., & Martin, J. B. (1983). A polymorphic DNA marker genetically linked to Huntington's disease. *Nature, 306,* 234–238.

Huntington's Disease Collaborative Research Group, Marcy E. MacDonald, *et al.* (1993). A novel gene containing a trinucleotide repeat that is expanded and unstable on Huntington's disease chromosomes. *Cell, 72,* 971–983.

Jonas, H. (1969). Philosophical reflections on experimenting with human subjects. In P. Freund (Ed.), *Experimentation with human subjects.* New York: George Braziller.

Kapp, M. B. (1994). Proxy decision making in Alzheimer disease research: Durable powers of attorney, guardianship and other alternatives. *Alzheimer Disease and Associated Disorders, 8*(Suppl. 4), 28–37.

Karlinsky, H., & Lennox, A. (1990). Assessment of competency of persons with Alzheimer's disease to provide consent for research. In J. M. Berg, H. Karlinsky, & F. Lowy (Eds.), *Alzheimer's disease research: Ethical and legal issues* (pp. 76–90). Toronto: Carswell.

Kerem, B.-S., Rommens, J. M., Buchanan, J. A., Markiewicz, D., Cox, T. K., Chakravarti, A., Buchwald, M., & Tsui, L.-C. (1989). Identification of the cystic fibrosis gene: Genetic analysis. *Science, 245,* 1073–1080.

Kevles, D. J. (1985). *In the name of eugenics.* Berkeley: University of California Press.

Kevles, D. J., & Hood, L. (1992). In D. J. Kevles & L. Hood (Eds.), *The code of codes: Scientific and social issues in the Human Genome Project* (pp. 300–328). Cambridge, MA: Harvard University Press.

Koenig, M., Hoffman, E. P., Bertelson, C. J., Monaco, A. P., Feener, C., & Kunkel, L. M. (1987). Complete cloning of the Duchenne muscular dystrophy (DMD) cDNA and preliminary genomic organization of the DMD gene in normal and affected individuals. *Cell, 50,* 509–517.

Krimsky, S. (1982). *Genetic alchemy: The social history of the recombinant DNA controversy.* Cambridge, MA: MIT Press.

Lawson, E. (1991, November 1). Personal notes from Cystic Fibrosis Studies Consortium Planning Meeting. Institute of Medicine.

Lee, W.-H., Bookstein, R., Hong, F., Young, L.-J., Shew, J.-Y., & Lee, E. Y.-H. P. (1987). Human retinoblastoma susceptibility gene: Cloning, identification, and sequence. *Science, 235,* 1394–1399.

Levi, J. (1991). Unproven AIDS therapies: The Food and Drug Administration and ddI. In K. E. Hanna (Ed.), *Biomedical politics* (pp. 9–37). Washington, DC: National Academy Press.

Li, F. P. (1992). Draft Recommendations on Predictive Testing for Germ Line p53 Mutations among Healthy Individuals. Presented to ELSI Working Group, February 10, 1992. Dana Farber Cancer Institute, Boston, January 31, 1992.

Lifton, R. J. (1986). *The Nazi doctors.* New York: Basic Books.

Marson, D. C., Schmitt, F. A., Ingram, K. K., & Harrell, L. (1994). Determining the competency of Alzheimer patients to consent to treatment and research. *Alzheimer Disease and Associated Disorders, 8*(Suppl. 4), 5–18.

Melnick, V. L., & Dubler, N. N. (Eds.). (1985). *Alzheimer's dementia: Dilemmas in clinical research.* Clifton, NJ: Humana Press.

National Center for Human Genome Research. (1990, October 8). NIH Collaboration Launches Research on Education and Counseling Related to Genetic Tests. Press release: Human Genome Project Progress. National Institutes of Health.

National Center for Human Genome Research, National Center for Nursing Research, National Institute of Child Health and Human Development and National Institute of Diabetes and Digestive and Kidney Diseases. (1991). RFA-HG-91-01. Studies of testing and counseling for cystic fibrosis mutations. *NIH Guide to Grants and Contracts, 20*(5 April), 5–6.

National Center for Human Genome Research. (1994). RFA: HG-94-01: Studies of genetic testing and counseling for heritable breast, ovarian and colon cancer risks. *NIH Guide to Grants and Contracts, 23*(4 February), 3–5.

National Commission for the Protection of Human Subjects of Biomedical and Behavioral Research, U.S. Department of Health, Education and Welfare. (1975). *Research on the fetus.* Washington, DC: U.S. Government Printing Office.

National Commission for the Protection of Human Subjects of Biomedical and Behavioral Research, U.S. Department of Health, Education and Welfare. (1976). *Research involving prisoners.* Washington, DC: U.S. Government Printing Office.

National Commission for the Protection of Human Subjects of Biomedical and Behavioral Research, U.S. Department of Health, Education and Welfare. (1977a). *Disclosure of research information under the Freedom of Information Act.* Washington, DC: U.S. Government Printing Office.

National Commission for the Protection of Human Subjects of Biomedical and Behavioral Research, U.S. Department of Health, Education and Welfare. (1977b). *Psychosurgery.* Washington, DC: U.S. Government Printing Office.

National Commission for the Protection of Human Subjects of Biomedical and Behavioral Research, U.S. Department of Health, Education and Welfare. (1977c). *Research involving children.* Washington, DC: U.S. Government Printing Office.

National Commission for the Protection of Human Subjects of Biomedical and Behavioral Research, U.S. Department of Health, Education and Welfare. (1978a). *The Belmont Report: Ethical principles and guidelines for the protection of human subjects of research.* Washington, DC: U.S. Government Printing Office. Reprinted in *Federal Register,* April 19, 1979.

National Commission for the Protection of Human Subjects of Biomedical and Behavioral Research, U.S. Department of Health, Education and Welfare. (1978b). *Ethical guidelines for the delivery of health services by DHEW.* Washington, DC: U.S. Government Printing Office.

National Commission for the Protection of Human Subjects of Biomedical and Behavioral Research, U.S. Department of Health, Education and Welfare. (1978c). *Institutional review boards.* Washington, DC: U.S. Government Printing Office.

National Commission for the Protection of Human Subjects of Biomedical and Behavioral Research. (1978d). *Research involving those institutionalized as mentally infirm* (DHEW Publication No. (OS) 78-0006). U.S. Department of Health, Education and Welfare.

National Commission for the Protection of Human Subjects of Biomedical and Behavioral Research, U.S. Department of Health, Education and Welfare. (1978e). *Special study: Implications of advances in biomedical and behavioral research.* Washington, DC: U.S. Government Printing Office.

National Research Council. (1988). *Mapping and sequencing the human genome. Washington, DC: National Academy Press.*

NCHGR Program Advisory Committee on the Human Genome. (1990, December 3). Resolution. National Center for Human Genome Research, National Institutes of Health.

NIH Workshop on Population Screening for the Cystic Fibrosis Gene. (1990, March 6). Statement. National Institutes of Health.

Office of Protection from Research Risks. (1993). *Protecting human research subjects: Institutional review board guidebook.* Bethesda: National Institutes of Health, U.S. Department of Health and Human Services.

Office of Science and Technology Policy. (1994, August 12). *Federal Register.*

Office of the Press Secretary, The White House. (1995, October 3). *Protection of human research subjects and creation of National Bioethics Advisory Commission.*

President's Commission for the Study of Ethical Problems in Medicine and Biomedical and Behavioral Research. (1981a). *Defining death.* Washington, DC: U.S. Government Printing Office.

President's Commission for the Study of Ethical Problems in Medicine and Biomedical and Behavioral Research. (1981b). *Protecting human subjects.* Washington, DC: U.S. Government Printing Office.

President's Commission for the Study of Ethical Problems in Medicine and Biomedical and Behavioral Research. (1982a). *Compenasating research injury.* Washington, DC: U.S. Government Printing Office.

President's Commission for the Study of Ethical Problems in Medicine and Biomedical and Behavioral Research. (1982b). *Making health care decisions* (with Vol. 2 and 3 appendices). Washington, DC: U.S. Government Printing Office.

President's Commission for the Study of Ethical Problems in Medicine and Biomedical and Behavioral Research. (1982c). *Splicing life.* Washington, DC: U.S. Government Printing Office.

President's Commission for the Study of Ethical Problems in Medicine and Biomedical and Behavioral Research. (1982d). *Whistleblowing in biomedical research.* Washington, DC: U.S. Government Printing Office.

President's Commission for the Study of Ethical Problems in Medicine and Biomedical and Behavioral Research. (1983a). *Deciding to forego life-sustaining treatment.* Washington, DC: U.S. Government Printing Office.

President's Commission for the Study of Ethical Problems in Medicine and Biomedical and Behavioral Research. (1983b). *Implementing human research regulations.* Washington, DC: U.S. Government Printing Office.

President's Commission for the Study of Ethical Problems in Medicine and Biomedical and Behavioral Research. (1983c). *Screening and counseling for genetic conditions.* Washington, DC: U.S. Government Printing Office.

President's Commission for the Study of Ethical Problems in Medicine and Biomedical and Behavioral Research. (1983d). *Securing access to health care.* Washington, DC: U.S. Government Printing Office.

President's Commission for the Study of Ethical Problems in Medicine and Biomedical and Behavioral Research. (1983e). *Summing up.* Washington, DC: U.S. Government Printing Office.

Proctor, R. N. (1988). *Racial hygiene: Medicine under the Nazis.* Cambridge, MA: Harvard University Press.

Ramsey, P. (1970). *The patient as person.* New Haven, CT: Yale University Press.

Rich, D. P., Anderson, M. P., Gregory, R. J., Cheng, S. H., Paul, S., Jefferson, D. M., McCann, J. D., Klinger, K. W., Smith, A. E., & Welsh, M. J. (1990). Expression of cystic fibrosis transmembrane conductance regulator corrects defective chloride channel regulation in cystic fibrosis airway epithelial cells. *Nature, 347,* 358–363.

Riordan, J. R., Rommens, J. M., Kerem, B.-S., Alon, N., Rozmahel, R., Grzelczak, Z., Zielenski, J., Lok, S., Plavsic, N., Chou, J.-L., Drumm, M. L., Iannuzzi, M. C., Collins, F. S., & Tsui, L.-C., (1989). Identification of the cystic fibrosis gene: Cloning and characterization of complementary DNA. *Science, 245,* 1066–1072.

Roberts, L. (1990). Cystic fibrosis pilot projects go begging. *Science, 250,* 1076–1077.

Roberts, L. (1993). Whither the ELSI Program? *Hastings Center Report, 23*(November–December), 5.

Rommens, J. M., Iannuzzi, M. C., *et al.,* (1989). Identification of the cystic fibrosis gene: Chromosome walking and jumping. *Science, 245,* 1059–1065.

Royer, B., Kunkel, L., Monaco, A., Goff, S., Newburger, P., Baehner, R., Cole, F., Curnutte, J., & Orkin, S. (1987). Cloning the gene for an inherited human disorder—chronic granulomatous disease—on the basis of its chromosomal location. *Nature, 322,* 32–38.

Simpson, S. G. (1993). Bipolar mood disorder. In M. S. Frankel & A. H. Teich (Eds.), *Ethical and legal issues in pedigree research* (pp. 39–63). Washington, DC: American Association for the Advancement of Science.

Thomson, E., & Drell, D. (1995, February 6). Presentations to the ELSI Working Group on the NIH and DOE ELSI grant portfolios, respectively. Holiday Inn, Bethesda.

Tsui, L.-C., Buchwald, M., *et al.,* (1985). Cystic fibrosis locus defined by a genetically linked polymorphic DNA marker. *Science, 230,* 1054–1057.

U.S. Congress. (1988, April). *Mapping our genes—Genome projects: How big? How fast?* Office of Technology Assessment (OTA-BA-373). Washington, DC: Government Printing Office; reprinted by Johns Hopkins University Press.

U.S. Congress (1993, June). *Biomedical ethics in US public policy* (OTA-BP-BBS-105). Background Paper. Office of Technology Assessment.

U.S. Department of Health, Education, and Welfare. (1978a). Proposed regulations on research involving those institutionalized as mentally disabled. *Federal Register, 43*(223), 53950–53956.

U.S. Department of Health, Education, and Welfare. (1978b). Protection of human subjects: Research involving those institutionalized as mentally infirm. *Federal Register, 43*(53), 11328–11358.

U.S. Senate. (1989, November 9). Human Genome Initiative. S. Hrg. 101-528. Subcommittee on Science, Technology and Space, Committee on Commerce, Science, and Transportation.

Wainwright, B. J., Scambler, P. J., Schmidtke, J., Watson, E. A., Law, H.-L., Farrall, M., Cooke, H. J., Eiberg, H., & Williamson, R. (1985). Localization of cystic fibrosis locus to human chromosome 7cen-q22. *Nature, 318,* 384–385.

Watson, J. D. (1988, September 26). NIH Press Conference: Appointment of James D. Watson to Head NIH Office of Human Genome Research. Bethesda: National Center for Human Genome Research; also available from the National Reference Center for Bioethics Literature, Georgetown University.

Weisburd, D. E. (Ed.). (1994). *The Journal,* Vol. 5, No. 1. Sacramento: California Alliance for the Mentally Ill.

White House. (1994, December 2). Statement by the President on NIH Recommendation Regarding Human Embryo Research. US Newswire. White House Press Office.

White, R., Woodward, S., Leppert, M., O'Connell, P., Hoff, M., Herbst, J., Lalouel, J.-M., Dean, M., & Vande Woude, G. (1985). A closely linked genetic marker for cystic fibrosis. *Nature, 318,* 382–384.

Wilfond, B. S., Fost, N. (1990, November 9). *Cystic fibrosis heterozygote detection: The introduc-
    tion of genetic testing into clinical practice.* Program in Medical Ethics, University of
    Wisconsin, presentation to ELSI Working Group. Revised versions of this paper were
    published in the *Journal of the American Medical Association, 263,* 2777–2783, 1991; and
    Milbank Quarterly, 70, 629–659, 1992.
Wilfond, B. S., & Nolan, K. (1993). National policy development for the clinical application
    of genetic diagnostic techniques. *Journal of the American Medical Association, 270,*
    2948–2954.

About the Authors

Mary Ann Beall

Mary Ann Beall is a mental health consumer who has been able to begin recovery in the last five years. She is an advocate and in 1993 won a Victory Award. She is Vice President for Administration of the Virginia Mental Health Consumers Association, serves on the Executive Committee of the Virginia Alliance for the Mentally Ill, and serves on the Board of Directors of the National Alliance for the Mentally Ill.

Robert Mullan Cook-Deegan, M.D.

Dr. Cook-Deegan, from the National Academy of Sciences, was Director of the Division of Biobehavioral Sciences and Mental Disorders at the Institute of Medicine from 1991 through 1994. He worked for the National Center for Human Genome Research from 1989 to 1990, after serving as Acting Executive Director of the Biomedical Ethics Advisory Committee of the U.S. Congress (1988–1989). Before that, he worked for the Office of Technology Assessment. In 1994 his book *The Gene Wars: Science, Politics, and the Human Genome* was published (New York: Norton). He received his bachelor's degree in chemistry, magna cum laude, in 1975 from Harvard College, and his M.D. degree from the University of Colorado in 1979.

Stephen V. Faraone, Ph.D.

Stephen V. Faraone earned a Ph.D. in psychology from the University of Iowa and completed postdoctoral training in psychiatric epidemiology and genetics at Brown Medical School. He is currently Associate Professor at Harvard Medical School's Department of Psychiatry at the Massachusetts Mental Health Center and Director of Research for the Pediatric Psychopharmacology Unit at Massachusetts General Hospital. Dr. Faraone is Associate Editor of *Neuropsychiatric Genetics* and maintains a research program in the epidemiology and genetics of schizophrenia, mood disorders, and attention-deficit hyperactivity disorder.

Irving I. Gottesman, Ph.D.

Irving I. Gottesman is the Sherrell J. Aston Professor of Psychology and Professor of Pediatrics (Genetics) at the University of Virginia in Charlottesville. Formerly, he was Professor of Psychiatric Genetics in the Departments of Psychiatry and of Genetics and Cell Biology at Washington University School of Medicine in St. Louis (1980–1985). He has worked in the areas of clinical psychology and human behavioral genetics since 1958 while then a graduate student at the University of Minnesota. His research in the United Kingdom with the late James Shields, using twins suffering from schizophrenia, has earned numerous honors and prizes, including an election to Honorary Fellow Royal College of Psychiatrists, the Stanley Dean Award for Schizophrenia Research, the Hoffheimer Prize, and the Kurt Schneider Prize. He is past president of both the Behavior Genetics Association and the Society for Research in Psychopathology.

Laura Lee Hall, Ph.D.

Laura Lee Hall is the Director of Research for the National Alliance for the Mentally Ill (NAMI). At NAMI since April, 1995, she is developing a policy and services research capacity in-house, to support their advocacy mission. Prior to joining NAMI, Laura was a senior analyst at the congressional Office of Technology Assessment, where she directed and authored several studies relevant to mental illness policy. She graduated magna cum laude from St. Francis College, Loretto, Pennsylvania, in 1983, where she majored in biology and minored in French. She received her doctoral degree in neuroscience from the Uniformed Services University for the Health Sciences, Bethesda, Maryland, in 1988, and held a postdoctoral fellowship at the National Institutes of Health through 1989.

Kay Redfield Jamison, Ph.D.

Kay Redfield Jamison is Professor of Psychiatry at the Johns Hopkins University School of Medicine. She is author of *Touched With Fire: Manic-Depressive Illness and the Artistic Temperament, An Unquiet Mind: A Memoir of Moods and Madness,* and coauthor of the standard medical text about manic-depressive illness. The latter was chosen in 1990 as the Most Outstanding Book in Biomedical Sciences by the American Association of Publishers. She is also the author of more than eighty scientific publications about mood disorders, suicide, psychotherapy, and lithium. Dr. Jamison, formerly the director of the UCLA Affective Disorders Clinic, was selected as the UCLA Woman of Science and is listed in *Best Doctors in the United States.* She is a member of the National Advisory Council for Human Genome Research, as well as the clinical director for the Dana Consortium on the Genetic Basis of Manic-Depressive Illness. She is also the executive producer and writer for a series of award-winning public television specials about manic-depressive illness and the arts.

Janet E. Johnson, M.D.

Dr. Johnson is Schizophrenia Research Fellow in the Department of Psychiatry, College of Physicians & Surgeons, Columbia University, where she pursues research interests in the genetics of schizophrenia, genetic counseling for neuropsychiatric disorders, and the ethical implications of the "new genetics" for psychiatric disease. She received her undergraduate education at the University of Missouri, Columbia, graduating with distinction in 1985. She received her doctorate at Missouri, her residency training at Tulane University Medical Center, and has been at Columbia since 1994.

Charles A. Kaufmann, M.D.

Dr. Kaufmann is Associate Professor in the Department of Psychiatry, College of Physicians & Surgeons, Columbia University, where he directs one of three national collaborating sites searching for major genes in schizophrenia as part of the NIMH Genetics Initiative. He also codirects the Schizophrenia Developing Clinical Research Center at Columbia (a center engaged in identifying genetic and epigenetic factors in the development of schizophrenia) and heads the Laboratory of Molecular Neurobiology at the New York State Psychiatric Institute (a laboratory devoted to the isolation of neuropsychiatric disease-relevant genes). Dr. Kaufmann received his undergraduate education in physics at MIT, graduating with highest distinction. He received his doctorate at Columbia, his residency training at Cornell's Payne Whitney Clinic, and spent five years as a Senior Staff Fellow in the Neuropsychiatry Branch, Intramural Research Program, NIMH, before returning to Columbia in 1986 for a postdoctoral fellowship in molecular biology with Dr. Eric Kandel. He has remained at Columbia ever since.

Herbert Pardes, M.D.

Dr. Pardes is Vice President for Health Sciences and Dean of the Faculty of Medicine at Columbia University. Former Director of the National Institute of Mental Health, trained as a psychiatrist, psychoanalyst, and researcher, he has chaired psychiatry departments at Downstate, Colorado, and Columbia. His background is broad: educator, administrator, researcher. He is past president of the American Psychiatric Association and the American Association of Chairmen of Departments of Psychiatry. He is Chairman of the Council of Deans of the Association of American Medical Colleges (AAMC) and Chair-elect of the AAMC. He is a member of the Insitute of Medicine.

Robert Plomin, Ph.D.

Robert Plomin is MRC Research Professor at the Institute of Psychiatry in London, where he is Deputy Director of the Social, Genetic and Developmental Psychiatry Research Centre. His research has focused on quantitative genetic approaches (i.e., twin and family studies) to behavioral development, although he is now most interested in using molecular genetics to investigate quantitative genetic problems at the interface between nature and nurture. His most recent book is *Genetics and Experience: The Interplay between Nature and Nurture* (Sage Publications, 1994).

Ming T. Tsuang, M.D., Ph.D., D.Sc., FRCPsych.

Dr. Tsuang is internationally known for his studies of the psychiatric epidemiology, nosology, and genetics of schizophrenia and mood disorders. Subsequent to receiving an M.D. degree from National Taiwan University, he earned his Ph.D. in psychiatry and D.Sc. in epidemiology and genetics at the Institute of Psychiatry, University of London. Currently, Dr. Tsuang is Stanley Cobb Professor of Psychiatry at Harvard Medical School, Superintendent and Head, Harvard Department of Psychiatry at the Massachusetts Mental Health Center, and Director of the Institute of Psychiatric Epidemiology and Genetics jointly sponsored by the Harvard Schools of Medicine and Public Health. He is also Chairman of the Veterans Affairs Cooperative Linkage Study of Schizophrenia at the Brockton/West Roxbury VA Medical Center. In addition to being Editor of the journal *Neuropsychiatric Genetics,* he continues to pursue epidemiological and genetic studies of schizophrenia, mood disorders, and substance use disorders. In recognition of his distinguished clinical and research career, he was elected Fellow, the Royal College of Psychiatrists of the United Kingdom, and Member, Institute of Medicine of the U.S. National Academy of Sciences.

Index